# Principles of
# Healthcare
# Leadership

# Principles of Healthcare Leadership

## BERNARD J. HEALEY

AUPHA

Health Administration Press, Chicago, Illinois

Association of University Programs in Health Administration, Washington, DC

Your board, staff, or clients may also benefit from this book's insight. For more information on quantity discounts, contact the Health Administration Press Marketing Manager at (312) 424-9450.

22   21   20   19   18        5   4   3   2   1

**Library of Congress Cataloging-in-Publication Data**
Names: Healey, Bernard J., 1947– author.
Title: Principles of healthcare leadership / Bernard J. Healey.
Description: Chicago, Illinois : Health Administration Press ; Washington, DC
    : Association of University Programs in Health Administration, [2018] |
    Includes bibliographical references and index.
Identifiers: LCCN 2017018677 (print) | LCCN 2017012031 (ebook) | ISBN
    9781567938937 (ebook) | ISBN 9781567938944 (xml) | ISBN 9781567938951
    (epub) | ISBN 9781567938968 (mobi) | ISBN 9781567938920 (print : alk. paper)
Subjects: LCSH: Health services administration—United States. |
    Leadership—United States.
Classification: LCC RA971 (print) | LCC RA971 .H3835 2018 (ebook) | DDC
    362.17/3068—dc23
LC record available at https://lccn.loc.gov/2017018677

Acquisitions editor: Jennette McClain; Project manager: Joyce Dunne; Cover designer: James Slate; Layout: PerfecType

Found an error or a typo? We want to know! Please e-mail it to hapbooks@ache.org, mentioning the book's title and putting "Book Error" in the subject line.

For photocopying and copyright information, please contact Copyright Clearance Center at www.copyright.com or at (978) 750-8400.

Health Administration Press
A division of the Foundation of the American
    College of Healthcare Executives
One North Franklin Street, Suite 1700
Chicago, IL 60606-3529
(312) 424-2800

Association of University Programs
    in Health Administration
1730 M Street, NW
Suite 407
Washington, DC 20036
(202) 763-7283

I would like to dedicate this new book to my wonderful grandson, John Bryan Healey. His birth gave me a desire to grow again.

# BRIEF CONTENTS

# DETAILED CONTENTS

# PREFACE

The major problems found in the current healthcare delivery system are cost escalation and diminished quality of healthcare services. Healthcare reform efforts over the past 50 years have yielded little success in overcoming these two enormous problems. In fact, numerous studies show that even while spending $3 trillion on healthcare services per year, the United States still ranks low in good health compared to other industrialized countries that spend far less. Many tools are being developed to lower healthcare costs and improve the quality of health services, but they will require skillful leadership for successful implementation. Unfortunately, healthcare innovations and reform efforts may be doomed to failure unless leaders emerge who can guide the healthcare sector through this process of change.

Since 1900, the longevity of most Americans has increased, with the majority of individuals now expected to live into their 80s. But because of the current epidemic of chronic diseases and their complications, a large percentage of these individuals will experience a decrease in quality of life as they age. In response, the US healthcare system must provide improved healthcare at a lower cost. This remedy requires improved leadership in every part of the system along with the empowerment of those who deliver these services to their patients. It also calls for a movement to be undertaken to shift organizational structures in healthcare from a bureaucratic management structure to a decentralized organizational framework.

To meet the current and future challenges in healthcare delivery, an immediate need is seen for leadership development for all employees. These leaders must rely less on their position power and more on their expertise and interpersonal skills to improve the quality of healthcare services. The old, bureaucratic US healthcare delivery system must be replaced by an organic form of shared power and responsibility that encourages the emergence of creativity and innovation to meet the demands of all stakeholders in that system. This transition is one reason this text devotes a large portion of its space to creativity and innovation in the delivery of healthcare services.

The US system of healthcare needs to be reorganized to improve productivity, which will eventually result in reduced costs for improved care for many consumers. As more providers enhance their performance, others will follow to remain competitive. The secret, then, for US healthcare organizations to survive, and even exploit, the changing healthcare environment is to hire and retain individuals who have the capacity to lead—rather than manage—their employees to deliver extraordinary services to their patients daily. This healthcare management text aims to elevate current and future leaders to new levels of knowledge, as seen among the most successful service delivery organizations in the world.

## About This Book

*Principles of Healthcare Leadership* is a comprehensive discussion surrounding the need for skillful leadership in US healthcare facilities. In addition, it covers the leadership styles found in organizations throughout the world. The book is composed of five parts:

- Introduction to Leadership in Healthcare
- Leadership Skills
- Organizational Culture Building
- Leading People in Healthcare Delivery
- Leadership Case Studies

Parts I through IV contain 11 chapters, each covering a separate aspect of knowledge required for healthcare leaders, all of whom are facing a turbulent environment of constant disruption. Part V constitutes five case studies that provide learning experiences through which students may practice the leadership skills presented in the preceding chapters. Each case begins with an explanation of a leadership issue in healthcare delivery, then describes a hypothetical use of the case information, and finally poses questions about the case and its application to the students.

The book was written to convey and fulfill the need both for current managers to develop new skills and for those planning to enter management positions to obtain these essential skills. They include leadership training in the empowerment of all health services employees to improve the quality of care they provide and the health outcomes for the population.

Additional skills required for the healthcare manager include

- change management and conflict management techniques,
- culture building,
- quality improvement skills,
- communication skills, and
- an appreciation for team building and collaboration.

This book shares with the reader the value of developing innovation skills in both managers and lower-level employees in healthcare facilities. In fact, the concept of entrepreneurship is covered at great length with the intent to move healthcare managers toward a decentralized and creative approach to healthcare facilities management.

The authors are aware of the need to include the physician in the discussion of change management, so a chapter on physician management—written by a physician—is included in this text. The book concludes with a chapter on future management challenges in health services delivery and suggested responses to these challenges.

---

## Instructor Resources

This book's Instructor Resources include an instructor's manual, a test bank, and PowerPoint slides for each chapter in this text. The instructor's manual includes an overview of each chapter and the answers to all the end-of-chapter discussion questions. The test bank is composed of true-or-false, multiple-choice, and essay questions as well as potential answers for these questions. Ten PowerPoint slides accompany each chapter to help guide instructors for each lecture.

For the most up-to-date information about this book and its Instructor Resources, visit ache.org/HAP and browse for the book's title or author name.

This book's Instructor Resources are available to instructors who adopt this book for use in their course. For access information, please e-mail hapbooks@ache.org.

# INTRODUCTION

The US healthcare system is experiencing massive changes in response to numerous environmental shifts that have been growing in intensity over the past several decades. Emanuel (2014) points out that our system of healthcare was not designed to be the inefficient, resource-consuming industry it has become. The inefficiencies resulted from the many poor decisions made early in the development of the care delivery system and have led to enormous cost increases with limited improvement in the health of most Americans.

Healthcare dollars have been spent on activities determined by the providers of care to be necessary with little or no consideration of the value or outcomes resulting from those activities. Emanuel (2014) argues that approximately one third of healthcare expenditures are wasted, with some of the activities also capable of producing real harm for the patient. These inefficiencies require a newly skilled leadership base to emerge throughout the US healthcare delivery system to save it from bankruptcy.

Kotter (2014) argues that many US organizations have failed to develop leaders capable of moving toward a creative, innovation-based future. Some observers attribute this leadership shortage to the fact that numerous industries in the United States are still using a bureaucratic organizational structure to conduct business. A bureaucracy is usually operated by managers who are concerned with the present while paying little attention to the future.

This absence of exceptional leadership in many US healthcare organizations can be attributed in part to the use of bureaucratic models, featuring an outdated, top-down management structure. The bureaucratic structure must be replaced with an approach driven by empowered workers in partnership with the leaders using a flattened organizational structure. A report issued by the Institute of Medicine (IOM) in 2001, titled *Crossing the Quality Chasm: A New Healthcare System for the 21st Century,* outlines the need for a complete reinvention of the US healthcare system. This report is critical of that system, claiming that it is incapable of producing the quality of care Americans require unless major, wholesale changes are made. IOM (2001) found that the system fails to achieve most Americans' expectations given its expense. Those failures stem from its overly complex nature and lack, for the most part, of coordination of care. The report offers the following system redesign imperatives (IOM 2001):

- Reengineer care processes.
- Use information technologies effectively.
- Adopt knowledge and skills management expertise.
- Develop effective teams.
- Coordinate care across patient conditions, services, and sites of care over time.

Schimpff (2012) further argues that to reduce the cost and improve the quality of care requires a comprehensive effort to coordinate care for those with chronic diseases. These diseases, along with their complications, are the main cause of cost escalation in healthcare and of poor-quality outcomes for the patients who have one or more chronic diseases. In addition to enhanced coordination of care for chronic diseases, he calls for the elimination of wasteful tests that do little to improve health outcomes. To effect these recommended changes, healthcare organizations must develop leadership skills in not only their executives and managers but also their employees, including physicians.

Many large organizations struggle with the need to give up past business practices for new ways of doing business to succeed in the disruptive business world. Govindarajan (2016) presents a solution that allows most businesses today to move forward in this process by segmenting the concerns they face into three separate boxes: managing the present, escaping the past ways of doing things, and preparing for the future. To operationalize this process, organizations must seek and develop leaders who can guide an empowered followership in understanding and responding to the three-box solution.

In particular, Govindarajan (2016) recommends that leaders gain an improved understanding of "planned opportunism," the ability to exploit opportunities that allow an organization to prepare for future disruptions in the present. The exploitation of opportunities is discussed at length in chapter 4.

This and numerous other strategies are presented throughout the book to point out options for US healthcare delivery organizations that face crises, such as cost escalation and diminished quality, failed past practices, and environmental disruption. More about the contents of this book follows.

## The Importance of Skilled Leadership

In this book, the authors suggest that the only way to meet the most serious challenges facing the US healthcare delivery system, in both the short term and the long term, is through skilled leadership that is developed specifically to address these challenges using emerging best practices and tapping the existing relevant theories of leadership in healthcare. Part I begins by explaining the theories of leadership, attending in particular to the concept of power and influence necessary for strong leadership. It then moves to a discussion of leadership skills, including best practices and the applicability of entrepreneurship and creativity.

Part II delves into the various leadership styles, including transformational leadership and servant leadership.

In Part III, the authors present the entire process of culture building in an organization, explaining how culture develops, the role of trust and culture development, and the need to build a thick positive culture.

Part IV addresses the specific issues related to leading people in healthcare delivery. Special emphasis is placed on the leadership process, development of strategy, and management of conflict.

By way of case studies, part V offers a multifaceted discussion of leadership development and the future of leadership in healthcare delivery. It considers up-to-date examples concerning the external environment leaders face as they attempt to deal with what seems like daily change in their redesigned organizations.

# References

Emanuel, E. J. 2014. *Reinventing American Health Care*. New York: Public Affairs.

Govindarajan, V. 2016. *The Three Box Solution: A Strategy for Leading Innovation*. Boston: Harvard Business Review Press.

Institute of Medicine (IOM). 2001. *Crossing the Quality Chasm: A New Health System for the 21st Century*. Washington, DC: National Academies Press.

Kotter, J. P. 2014. *Accelerate: Building Strategic Agility for a Faster-Moving World*. Boston: Harvard Business Review Press.

Schimpff, S. C. 2012. *The Future of Health Care Delivery: Why It Must Change and How It Will Affect You*. Washington, DC: Potomac.

# INTRODUCTION TO LEADERSHIP IN HEALTHCARE

# THE FUTURE OF LEADERSHIP IN HEALTHCARE

Bernard J. Healey

## Learning Objectives

After completing this chapter, the reader should be able to

- identify the major challenges facing the US healthcare delivery system and potential solutions to them,
- understand the need for change in healthcare delivery,
- understand the role of leadership in preparing the organization to meet the future challenges, and
- recognize the need for healthcare leaders and followers to work together toward solving the many US healthcare issues at hand.

## Key Terms and Concepts

- Affordable Care Act (ACA)
- Comparative effectiveness research (CER)
- Cost–benefit analysis
- Cost-effectiveness analysis
- Fee-for-service
- MRSA (methicillin-resistant *Staphylococcus aureus*)
- Paradigm shift
- Pay for performance (P4P)
- Psychological trap
- Resource trap

## Introduction

No one can predict with certainty the future of healthcare in the United States. Despite this fact, some researchers and authors have come out with their own predictions concerning the healthcare delivery system over the next ten years.

The only certainty is that the continuing escalation of healthcare costs, along with the diminishing quality of healthcare services, is not sustainable for much longer. Few individuals seem happy with the current healthcare system, including those who purchase healthcare services and those who deliver these services. In addition, the healthcare industry is ripe for disruption by low-cost providers who concentrate on giving consumers what they want in terms of healthcare delivery at a lower price. The healthcare industry is in the process of major change, and that shift is descending quickly.

In his book *Disrupt You: Master Personal Transformation, Seize Opportunity, and Thrive in the Era of Endless Innovation,* Samit (2015) points out the classic traps of corporate success covered by Vijay Govindarajan in his research. As demonstrated in Samit's book, Govindarajan (2016) describes them as a resource trap, a management psychological trap, and a failure to plan for the future. These traps are all wide open, ready to capture unaware staff, and are found in many healthcare organizations despite numerous warnings to root them out. Some healthcare organizations have already been disrupted by other companies taking advantage of these traps to the point that the organizations must file for bankruptcy.

**Resource trap**
A situation prohibitive to growth in which organizations invest scarce resources in old systems that do not work.

The **resource trap** can be seen in organizations that continue to invest scarce resources in old systems rather than looking long and hard at what the future requires. One example is the organization that continues to invest in buildings that the future healthcare organization may not even require, a scenario being played out in many healthcare systems expanding emergency departments (EDs) with little consideration of changing reimbursement procedures that may not favor utilization of the ED.

**Psychological trap**
A management barrier to progress that occurs when an organization holds on to the past as the default option.

The second trap, known as a management **psychological trap**, is common in healthcare systems that hold onto the ways activities and processes have been performed in the past. Healthcare administrators spend countless hours in so-called planning meetings and talk about past successes and how they need to be continued into the future. The current turbulence in the US healthcare environment is disrupting almost every part of the delivery system, and past successes do not ensure that past processes will continue to work.

The third trap mentioned by Govindarajan (2016) is the inability to plan for an evolving future. In healthcare, this trap is evident as many current administrators have failed to realize the future role for healthcare providers in the prevention of illness. Instead, they continue to focus on treating chronic diseases and their complications after they occur. To thrive under a value-based reimbursement model, healthcare organizations must design a strategy to prevent the complications of chronic diseases from developing and deploy resources to prevent chronic diseases from occurring in the first place.

Responding to these three management traps, especially as they relate to concerns of chronic diseases, requires a **paradigm shift** for most healthcare organizations. They often have failed to view the prevention of disease as their primary responsibility, being more interested in—and rewarded for—curing disease after it has occurred. Prior to the shift from volume- to value-driven incentives, organizations made little effort to keep people well because of the way the reimbursement system was structured and the fact that people usually consider visiting a provider only when they are ill. These factors led to a reimbursement system whereby providers were paid for services rendered, known as fee-for-service (discussed later in the book). Furthermore, medical education is centered on treating curable diseases, mainly by prescribing one or more drugs. Though well-intended and often effective in making patients healthy, a new emphasis should be placed on an illness prevention paradigm throughout the US healthcare system.

**Paradigm shift**
A change in the way one thinks about how to proceed through a process or design an activity.

Once the healthcare organization leaders and staff get serious about keeping people healthy rather than having to treat illness, or even allowing the population to get sick, a reduction in the cost of healthcare and an improvement in their population's health status should occur. Those who are responsible for reimbursing providers of care—payers—also need to shift the reimbursement structure from incentives to achieve the cure to those that reward prevention of disease. The time for discussing the need for prevention programs is over; healthcare leaders now must make the changes. This change can occur, through strong leadership throughout healthcare organizations, by altering the way healthcare is provided to consumers.

## The Changing Healthcare Environment

Most health policymakers agree that the real cause of both cost escalation and diminished quality of healthcare services is the epidemic of chronic diseases and their complications. One important component of solving this complex problem is enhanced leadership, along with empowered followers, that supports creativity and innovation in the development, implementation, and evaluation of health education initiatives among organizations throughout the United States. The US healthcare system has no capacity for separate operational or professional silos, nor for professions' desire to hang onto power as if their existence depended on it.

The main question that needs to be answered by healthcare researchers is what changes in the delivery system will occur over the next several years because of the shifting healthcare environment. Numerous experts in health policy research have attempted to answer this question, but agreement on the results is lacking. Some experts predict the system will go into a crisis mode, seeing no end in sight to escalation of costs and lowered quality of care. Others view all the changes as a tremendous opportunity to build a new system of healthcare delivery that contains costs while improving quality. This new system of healthcare delivery, if designed properly, should also result in a healthier population.

**Affordable Care Act (ACA)**
Signed into law in 2010, the act seeks to increase the quality and availability of healthcare coverage for most Americans.

According to Emanuel (2014), an architect of the **Affordable Care Act (ACA)**, six megatrends will directly result from the 2010 legislation, assuming the ACA remains intact during the Donald Trump administration. These shifts should be evident following 2020 and include the following:

- A change in the care of chronic diseases and mental health care
- Hospital closures
- Major changes to medical education
- A change in the role of health insurance companies
- The end of employer-financed health insurance
- The end of cost escalation

Each megatrend is explored further in the paragraphs that follow.

One might view these six trends as resembling dominoes ready to collapse. If we are unable to reduce significantly the complications from chronic diseases and their attendant costs, these diseases may bankrupt the United States. This situation calls for significant changes to address chronic diseases, including mental health issues.

The use of hospitals as a center for healthcare delivery is an outdated concept long overdue for change. Hospitals suffer from the so-called cost disease found in nearly every sector of the healthcare delivery system. This author is confident that the expansion of chronic diseases will be reversed, and when that happens, overall hospital census will drop. However, hospitals continue to expand capacity in almost identical fashion to colleges, which continue to purchase real estate while experiencing drops in enrollment.

A change in the way physicians are educated is similarly overdue, but such shifts face tremendous resistance. Physicians receive redundant medical training but little education in the prevention of disease and team leadership. As reimbursement systems change from fee-for-service to payment for outcomes, physicians need to expand their knowledge of proven prevention techniques that will be necessary to reduce the complications arising from long-present chronic disease.

To realize Emanuel's (2014) projected changes to the insurance industry and the employer's role, a serious discussion regarding third-party payers must take place, beginning with ways to reduce the costs of healthcare delivery and improve the quality of care delivered. These goals are not being achieved by the prevailing system, whereby insurance companies collect money from employers and then reimburse providers for activities that may or may not improve the health of US populations. The discussion must include the employers who are paying the ever-increasing bill, currently written off as an expense of doing business.

Much discourse in recent years has concerned the creative destruction of the US health insurance industry. The providers of health insurance have not used their market power as an incentive to demand better quality and lower prices from the providers they essentially employ. Instead, a steady trend has been seen of reduced payments and increased denials of care for their consumers. A much better strategy is to motivate providers to provide the right care rather than denying care—resulting in the final megatrend, an end to healthcare cost escalation.

Emanuel's (2014) predictions seem accurate considering the currently turbulent healthcare environment. In this textbook, we use these predictions as background for proposing how the US healthcare system can deal with the major problems discussed.

## Changing Reimbursement Methods

One major reason for the continued cost escalation in healthcare delivery is the way providers of care are reimbursed for their services. It is not the intent of this chapter to explain the history of healthcare finance or provide an overview of the many reimbursement terms that make payment for healthcare services so different from the financing used in the payment for most goods and services in the US economy. Instead, the focus is on demonstrating how the reimbursement methods for healthcare services will change and how these changes will affect the future of US healthcare delivery.

As mentioned previously, the historical approach to paying providers has been on a **fee-for-service** basis. The problem with this payment mechanism is that it encourages providers to offer more care than necessary, bringing little value and perhaps even harm to the patient. In essence, it allows the care provider to create her own demand for healthcare.

To eliminate this so-called perverse incentive, a movement must take place to reimburse providers for healthy patient outcomes. To be successful, this move to performance-based reimbursement, or **pay for performance (P4P)**, requires healthcare providers to work *with* their patients by offering

**Fee-for-service**
A healthcare services reimbursement model whereby providers are paid for the quantity of services offered.

**Pay-for-performance (P4P)**
A payment system that offers providers of care financial incentives for achieving improved patient outcomes.

education about their health status and how to avoid high-risk health behaviors that result in chronic diseases and their complications. A great deal of physician–patient contact is necessary under this system.

With increased contact between physicians and patients comes increased payment to the provider. Even so, overall costs should eventually be reduced because of the positive impact this patient education is expected to have on population health.

If more than $3 trillion a year is expended in the United States on healthcare services, we should have a good idea of what services work best and what interventions in healthcare should not be reimbursed. This expectation is a main reason so much discussion has emerged about **comparative effectiveness research (CER)**.

**Comparative effectiveness research (CER)**
Studies that evaluate the benefits, harms, and effectiveness of different treatment options.

### The Role of Comparative Effectiveness Research

Feldstein (2015) notes that health economists have long been interested in using economic analysis to decide how scarce healthcare resources should be used. The most popular forms of economic analysis are **cost-effectiveness analysis** and **cost–benefit analysis**. Simply stated, the costs of medical procedures are compared with the benefits that result from the use of those procedures. If adopted, economic analysis would help identify and eliminate approximately $1 trillion a year worth of waste on unnecessary and potentially harmful medical procedures.

**Cost-effectiveness analysis**
An economics-focused process for comparing the cost of an intervention to its effectiveness.

Encouraging the elimination of $1 trillion in wasteful healthcare services through economic analysis is a compelling idea. But how does an organization determine what represents waste in the delivery of healthcare services? The answer is CER.

**Cost–benefit analysis**
An economics-focused process for comparing the strengths and weaknesses of alternative choices in healthcare provision.

Feldstein (2015) indicates that more than $1 billion was allocated to CER in 2009 as part of the American Recovery and Reinvestment Act, and an additional $3 billion was made available for CER through the ACA. CER has helped decision makers determine the cost and value of treatment options by testing the effectiveness of medical procedures and seeking less expensive alternatives for achieving a positive outcome.

An early attempt at evaluating medical care was conducted in 1967 by John Wennberg, at the Institute for Health Policy and Clinical Practice of Dartmouth College. Wennberg (2010) analyzed medical data to determine how well hospitals and physicians were performing. He found tremendous variation in every aspect of healthcare delivery—practice patterns, types of medical tests ordered, and types or numbers of surgeries performed—depending on geographic location. Worth noting is that such variation continues throughout the United States.

For example, exhibit 1.1 offers a comparison of total reimbursement per decedent for treatment during the final two years of life at several US academic medical centers. As seen in the exhibit, wide variations are evident in each measure. Feldstein (2015) argues that this type of information can provide a great service to the US healthcare system by helping to determine the effectiveness of treatments and medicines. This knowledge can then be shared broadly through the practice of evidence-based medicine to improve the quality of care delivered.

To complement the promise of CER and ensure the system's ability to control healthcare costs, an organized effort is needed to find accurate data with which to prove the value, or lack of value, of treatment regimens for the vast majority of health issues. That both positive and negative implications are inherent in the use of CER for reimbursement determinations should not stop this important discussion from continuing. Discovering the best way to handle different medical conditions helps guarantee quality service to all US residents at a cost all can afford.

**EXHIBIT 1.1**
Medicare Spending per Decedent During the Last Two Years of Life (Deaths Occurring in 2010), Select Academic Medical Centers

| Academic Medical Center | Inpatient Reimbursements per Decedent | Hospital Days per Decedent | Reimbursements per Day |
|---|---|---|---|
| Johns Hopkins Hospital | $88,750 | 26.8 | $3,311 |
| Ronald Reagan UCLA Medical Center | $78,196 | 28.5 | $2,740 |
| University of Maryland Medical Center | $78,156 | 24.9 | $3,135 |
| Hahnemann University Hospital | $69,304 | 36.3 | $1,909 |
| Massachusetts General Hospital | $51,385 | 26.7 | $1,925 |
| Cleveland Clinic Foundation | $46,100 | 25.5 | $1,807 |
| Mayo Clinic–St. Mary's Hospital | $36,411 | 17.5 | $2,082 |
| Scott & White Memorial Hospital | $32,354 | 15.2 | $2,127 |

*Source:* Reprinted from Feldstein (2015). Data from the Dartmouth Institute for Health Policy & Clinical Practice.

## Measuring the Quality of Healthcare

In recent years, the Institute of Medicine (IOM) has raised concerns about the quality of healthcare services in the United States. It has published several research-based reports concerning quality indexes along with numerous recommendations for how to improve healthcare quality (e.g., IOM 2000). Among the most serious quality issues being addressed are medication errors and hospital-acquired infections.

Claxton and colleagues (2015) present a number of reasons for concern regarding diminished quality in health services delivery. Some of these reasons are discussed next.

### Healthcare Services Are Vital for Everyone

When one becomes ill, one usually is unable to work and enjoy life. In this situation, there is no substitute for healthcare services. The individual in need of healthcare wants the best care possible and generally is not concerned about the price of that care. Because most US healthcare consumers do not have a medical background, they tend to evaluate their experience on the basis of service criteria: the amount of time they have to wait, the length of their visit with the physician, how well they are treated by the organization's staff, whether their health situation improved as a result of their visit to the healthcare facility, and so on.

### Healthcare Services Are Very Expensive

Two major problems are associated with the cost of healthcare. The first is that most consumers have been insulated from healthcare cost escalation because their employer has paid much of the bill. The second, more recent problem is that employers are accepting less responsibility for healthcare coverage. As a result, consumers are now exposed to the implications of healthcare cost. They may even come to recognize that waste occurs in the healthcare delivery system and, because they now pay a larger portion of the bill, that waste directly affects their wallet.

### Healthcare Services Are Complex to Deliver

Healthcare services are complex and very difficult for the average consumer to understand, much less measure. Healthcare leaders need to make certain their staff understand the importance of communicating well and appropriately with consumers. In addition, leaders must clearly define all service offerings, including their risks and costs.

# How Leaders Can Meet the Major Healthcare Challenges

Meeting the major challenges faced by US healthcare organizations over the next several years requires strong leadership to implement solutions. These problems will not go away by themselves; they must be addressed by the leaders of hospitals and health systems using approaches such as those proposed later in this section. The solutions are not easy to implement, especially without a team approach.

Finally, organizations must be committed to full implementation of the solutions. They will require a long time to develop and implement, and an even longer time for improvements to be noticeable. However, the US healthcare system is running out of time. Recommended solutions to the aforementioned challenges are presented in the following sections.

### *Invest in Health Education Programs*

As mentioned earlier in this chapter, the primary cause of the escalation in healthcare costs every year is the epidemic of chronic diseases and their complications. According to Schimpff (2012), individuals' health behaviors are the major determinant of such disease. Health behaviors are learned, and they can be changed through health education programs.

An obvious starting point is to institute these programs as part of every patient encounter with a healthcare delivery system and make sure they include all providers of healthcare services. The provider's role has always been the missing link between the availability of health education material and that material being received and understood by the patient population. Bridging this gap may mark the ideal opportunity to tap the well-documented respect that most patients have for their physicians as the necessary ingredient to make health education initiatives work. According to Centers for Disease Control and Prevention (CDC 2002), many individuals do not understand the ramifications of a continuous practice of high-risk health behavior, and the message about this danger needs to be reinforced by the provider at every patient encounter.

This mandate is not on the physician alone to fulfill, however; it is a leadership issue for those in charge of healthcare organizations as well. The leader of the healthcare facility has the responsibility to deliver to customers the best healthcare possible. This duty entails making certain that all physicians working in the facility are making every effort to keep their patients healthy. Most physicians will gladly educate their patients if they are allotted appropriate time to do so. The leader's responsibility is to ensure that the time is made available for health education.

Not as obvious a step but just as important, the health education process should be included in the educational curriculum of every US school district, from preschool through high school. In addition, health education programs need to become a large part of the work environment. The workplace is an excellent location for sharing important health information that is necessary to prevent the development of chronic diseases and reduce the occurrence of their complications over time. One example of this concept is the number of companies that now make available to their employees a comprehensive collection of information about type 2 diabetes. This inexpensive health education effort can result in large payoffs if it helps prevent the expensive complications that can arise from type 2 diabetes over a long period.

### Invest in Population Health

A natural extension of health education initiatives is for healthcare facilities to accept the responsibility for achieving and maintaining a healthy population. White and Griffith (2016) point out that population health is concerned with ensuring that members of the community can function at the highest level possible with community resources. Exhibit 1.2 looks at the components required for a healthy community, demonstrating that costs rise as a population moves from the healthy state. This exhibit shows that optimum care is maximized with enhanced use of preventive services and ambulatory care.

White and Griffith (2016) point to three interrelated aspects of healthcare delivery that have directed the system to emphasize acute care and minimize the emphasis on preventive care:

- An emphasis on healthcare financing
- Compensation to providers
- Organizational responses

Each of these components is discussed in later chapters.

### Expand Programs to Prevent Errors and Infections

According to IOM (2000), from 44,000 to 98,000 of the 33 million individual patients hospitalized every year die, and many more hospitalized patients are beset by hospital-acquired infections because of poor-quality healthcare administered during their hospitalization. IOM (2000) also reports that between 2.9 and 3.7 percent of patients admitted to hospitals experience injury or death while under their care.

This is an important area of healthcare delivery requiring immediate intervention by the leader. It represents the worst outcome that could result from hospitalization of an ill patient. These medical mistakes are often referred to as "never events" because they should never happen, and it is

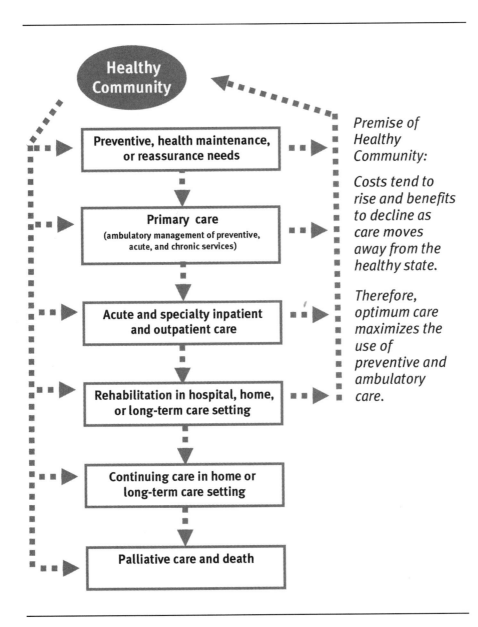

**EXHIBIT 1.2**
A Conceptual Model for Personal Services for Population Health

*Source:* Reprinted from White and Griffith (2016).

up to the leaders to institute procedures that make certain these mistakes become true never events.

Many reasons help explain the epidemic of medical errors experienced each year in medical facilities throughout the United States. IOM (2007) points out that the major reason for medical errors is a lack of communication or poor communication among providers of care. Patients commonly receive medical care from numerous providers simultaneously, and most often, some or all of those providers lack accurate and up-to-date medical information about their patients. Medication errors on a daily basis are a result.

A study completed by IOM in 2006 revealed that approximately 400,000 errors occur per year in hospitals, 800,000 errors occur in long-term care settings, and an additional 530,000 errors occur in Medicare patients visiting outpatient clinics for care. Improved communications among all employees not only make a positive difference in the costs of healthcare but also, and more important, improve the quality of care.

Nosocomial infections are healthcare-associated (or hospital-acquired) infections, meaning they are not present when an individual is admitted to a hospital but occur while the patient is being treated there as an inpatient, usually resulting from interaction with facility employees. In addition to being potentially deadly to the patient, these infections are expensive to treat and are subject to penalties by the Centers for Medicare & Medicaid Services if they require readmission of the patient. The CDC (2016) reports that 722,000 hospital-acquired infections occurred in 2011. These infections result in longer inpatient stays, higher mortality rates, and increased healthcare costs. They also lower the quality of care delivered by healthcare facilities and, ultimately, lead to loss of consumer trust in a hospital or health system.

Medical errors and hospital-acquired infections result from human or system errors and need to be dealt with through enhanced leadership. According to IOM (2000), the most common error found in hospitals involves administering drugs to patients. Every medication error alone adds approximately $5,000 to the cost of a hospital stay. Of highest concern, of course, is that on top of the monetary expense of slipshod medical care, patients and families—and the organization itself—must deal with any disability or the death of a patient who came to the hospital for medical help.

Hospital-acquired infections result from the housing of large numbers of patients together for an extended period. One well-known example of a hospital-acquired infection is methicillin-resistant *Staphylococcus aureus,*

**MRSA (methicillin-resistant *Staphylococcus aureus*)**
A type of staph bacteria that has become resistant to antibiotics.

better known as **MRSA.** MRSA has emerged as a major public health issue, despite the fact that many MRSA infections can be prevented through strong enforcement of sanitation techniques, such as a hand-washing protocol and requiring all medical personnel to use alcohol rubs before and after each patient contact.

One example of a leadership solution to a patient safety problem is found in Paul O'Neill's work reducing errors at ALCOA. As documented by Spear (2009), the number one priority outlined by O'Neill in his first meeting with staff after assuming the ALCOA CEO role was planned safety. O'Neill instituted a comprehensive strategy to eliminate accidents that included notification be delivered, within 24 hours of an accident at ALCOA, to O'Neill by the vice president of the section where the accident occurred.

This procedure let everyone in the organization know the CEO was making accident prevention a priority.

This rapid reporting of the accident was followed by a swarming of the accident and a written report generated as to its cause. Swarming accidents involves a complete investigation and a determination of cause by senior management staff and safety personnel. Resources were made available to develop prevention programs helping to ensure the same accident did not occur in the future. Once the information was gathered, it was shared throughout the organization. This strategy was successful in reducing injuries resulting from accidents from 2 to 0.07 percent, setting an industry-leading benchmark for large organizations (Spear 2009). At ALCOA, strong leadership solved a dangerous and costly problem that is found in many healthcare organizations.

### Invest in Healthcare Delivery Innovation

The vast majority of US healthcare organizations have adopted and maintain a bureaucratic organization run by managers concerned with operating an efficient organization. In this model, a system of checks and balances and rules and regulations is in place, supported by employees and enforced by a master's-degreed healthcare manager. While its intent is reasonable, this structure does not promote creativity or foster innovation, limiting its effectiveness.

Many start-up companies are moving to the fringes of healthcare delivery to disrupt the largest industry in the United States. Traditional healthcare organizations need to embrace the concept of entrepreneurship and intrapreneurship to bring creativity and innovation to all their segments. Such a major operational shift requires strong leadership not only from the designated leader but also from all of his employees. Kotter (2014) argues that an organization's leadership represents the major force necessary to mobilize employees to create what will likely amount to a new care delivery model. Healthcare organizations must reorganize their entire structure to create new ways of delivering healthcare to their customers.

No one can say what the new healthcare organization will look like once all of the changes are made. The only certainty is that the employees and the customers will be the driving forces if the organization is to remain in business and grow.

It is time for healthcare organizations to realize that they already have all the talent they need to solve most of their problems. The missing link in meeting the challenges of healthcare services delivery in the United States is leadership and empowered followership. Those leaders and empowered followers, once identified and enabled, must work to redesign their healthcare organizations to allow creativity to emerge. That creativity should allow these employees to take the risks necessary for creating a business environment that fosters intrapreneurship, in turn allowing the creation of new products and services.

Most healthcare organizations that take the time and effort to talk with their customers discover that what consumers want is courteous staff encounters—including with the physician—and less expensive services, less waste of their valuable time, and less paperwork than they currently endure. Increasingly, consumers will go elsewhere if they are not satisfied on these terms.

### Understand the New Healthcare Patient

Thus, the former patient of healthcare services has become the consumer of healthcare products and services. This consumer is now paying a significant portion of his healthcare bill, and thanks to the availability of information regarding health, he has become a well-informed consumer of medical care. In fact, every sign indicates that the consumer now wants to be part of the medical care decision-making process at every step of care.

Topol (2015) argues that patient-consumers know their bodies and have realized that no one has a greater interest in their good health than they have. They also demand to receive the same courteous treatment from their provider as they receive when they purchase any other product or service. According to Topol (2015), patient-consumers are tired of the way healthcare services are traditionally delivered and are sharing all of their frustrations on social media, such as Facebook and Twitter. In his book *The Patient Will See You Now*, for example, he shares numerous studies related to the problems that patients encounter with healthcare delivery across the country. According to his research, patients wait an average of 62 minutes to see a physician for a 7-minute visit, an unacceptable scenario. Patients are also upset with hospital-acquired infections and receiving a hospital bill they cannot understand or afford. As a result, they are becoming real consumers of healthcare and demanding accountability from their providers. They are uniting through their smartphones and social media and finding apps that provide them with the information necessary to become an informed consumer (Topol 2015).

This movement can be a positive shift for everyone involved in healthcare services delivery. For this positivity to be realized, the healthcare organization must realize that the patient is the most important part of the process of reinventing healthcare in the United States. The patient deserves care that involves the patient and family members in planning and decision making about the choices to be made (White and Griffith 2016).

### Make Incentives Work

Incentives are meant to motivate an individual to act or not act in a certain way. Economic incentives have been used seemingly since the beginning of time to motivate others toward achieving a goal. One prevailing approach to motivating healthcare employees has been to increase salaries or offer bonuses to increase production, resulting in increased profit for the employer. However, many of the incentives used in healthcare delivery are given to those who exhibit market power and influence and are represented by powerful interest groups.

A great deal of experimentation with incentives is needed to discover designs that encourage positive changes in the way healthcare services are provided. Employees motivated to eliminate the $1 trillion in waste experienced in healthcare annually, for example, could offer solutions to enhance the delivery of healthcare services if given the chance to address their specific areas of expertise.

Developing the right incentives will go a long way toward changing the US healthcare delivery system to reduce costs and improve quality. Incentives matter, but they can also produce bad behaviors. Healthcare leaders must learn as much as they can about what motivates followers to help effect the monumental change required.

Healthcare leaders also need to understand how incentives work toward the improvement of population health. As stated previously, the health of the population needs to be a responsibility of the entire community, including healthcare organizations. Once healthcare facilities and other community agencies begin to offer high-quality, effective health education information and materials, designing incentives to promote preventive care should not be difficult.

### *Invest in the Leadership Solution*

The days of ignoring the problems in the US healthcare delivery system are long gone, and solutions are needed now. In the currently turbulent reform era in healthcare, one solution that seems to make sense is to supplement strong leadership with empowered employees working hard to innovate the way healthcare services are delivered.

To be successful in this reform effort, they need to solve all of the related problems at the same time. The starting point in the leadership solution is to understand that management is not the same concept as leadership. Managers worry about efficiency in production, whereas leaders are concerned with future success for the organization and its employees or, as Kotter (2012) states, with organizing groups of people and preparing them to move into an improved future.

Joshi and colleagues (2014) point out that for healthcare leaders to influence others, they need strong leadership attributes and must know how and when to use them. The leadership solution requires the skills of being and doing outlined in exhibit 1.3. Here, the healthcare leader asks for a complete reframing of core values that shapes transformational leadership on a daily basis throughout the organization. Exhibit 1.3 explains what the leader must represent to her followers and presents several specific tasks that she needs to complete consistently.

The healthcare leader must be authentic and trustworthy while demonstrating humility as part of the position of authority. Followers look for their leaders to be "in love with" their work, exhibiting energy while focusing on results and building relationships with employees and customers.

Joshi and colleagues (2014) argue that improving the quality of the healthcare system requires leaders to work on the improvement of the entire system. To do so, the leader must gain a complete understanding of all aspects of delivering high-quality health services on a consistent basis. This expectation makes sense when we consider the interconnectedness of all we do in healthcare delivery. In particular, Joshi and colleagues point to interrelated activities that include setting direction; establishing the foundation of exemplary service; and building will, generating ideas, and executing change.

A critical aspect of this solution is a point we have already touched on: for all stakeholders to work together. Tett (2015) notes that the new world of work is integrated because of technology but has also become increasingly fragmented in terms of approaches to solving problems. He argues the silos that have developed and expanded in the twenty-first century are dangerous in this new world because, as people participate in fragmented groups, they

**EXHIBIT 1.3**
Individual Leadership: Being and Doing

| What Leaders Must Be (Examples) | What Leaders Must Know How to Do (Examples) |
|---|---|
| • An authentic embodiment of core values<br>• Trustworthy: consistent in thought, word, and deed<br>• In love with the work, rather than the position, of leadership<br>• Someone who adds energy to a team, rather than sucks it out<br>• Humble, but not insecure; able to say, "I was wrong"<br>• Focused on results, rather than popularity<br>• Capable of building relationships<br>• Passionately committed to the mission | • Understand the system context in which improvement work is being done<br>• Explain how the work of the team fits into the aims of the whole system<br>• Use and teach improvement methods<br>• Develop new leaders<br>• Explain and challenge the current reality<br>• Inspire a shared vision<br>• Enable others to act<br>• Model the way<br>• Encourage the heart (Kouzes and Posner 2003)<br>• Manage complex projects |

*Source:* Reprinted from Joshi et al. (2014).

remove their expertise from the knowledge base of every other group. These silos become protected, reducing communication among large groups of people attempting to solve similar problems.

## Summary

The most important question that needs to be answered by health policymakers and researchers working in healthcare seems to be what changes in our delivery system will occur over the next several years due to the changing healthcare environment. The current healthcare delivery system is in crisis thanks to all the disruption being caused by the escalation of healthcare costs and the diminished quality of healthcare services. These changes present a tremendous opportunity to build a new system of healthcare that reduces costs while improving the quality of services delivered.

The only solution to the many healthcare challenges may be the use of strong leadership supplemented with empowered employees working hard to innovate the way healthcare services are delivered. Healthcare leaders and their followers must understand that to be successful in this reform effort they need to solve all of the related problems at the same time. These problems reflect poor leadership and can be solved by the provision of informed and proactive leadership solutions.

The starting point in using the leadership solution to meet the challenges faced by healthcare organizations today is to understand that management is not leadership. Leadership is associated with great change, and it must take place in healthcare soon as possible, or many healthcare organizations will not be around in the long term.

## Discussion Questions

1. Name and explain some of the major changes that will occur in healthcare delivery over the next several years.
2. What are the classic traps of corporate success that need to be avoided by healthcare delivery systems as they respond to disruption?
3. Explain the ramifications for healthcare providers of the major changes being predicted by healthcare researchers and policymakers over the next decade.
4. Discuss the components found in the leadership solution for the challenges faced by US healthcare organizations.

# References

Centers for Disease Control and Prevention (CDC). 2016. "HAI Data and Statistics." Updated October 5. www.cdc.gov/hai/surveillance/.

———. 2002. "Behavioral Risk Factor Surveillance System Survey Data." Atlanta, GA: CDC.

Claxton, G., C. Cox, S. Gonzales, R. Kamal, and L. Levitt. 2015. "Measuring the Quality of Healthcare in the U.S." *Kaiser Family Foundation.* Published September 10. www.healthsystemtracker.org/insight/measuring-the-quality-of-healthcare-in-the-u-s/.

Emanuel, E. J. 2014. *Reinventing American Health Care.* New York: Public Affairs.

Feldstein, P. J. 2015. *Health Policy Issues: An Economic Perspective,* 6th ed. Chicago: Health Administration Press.

Govindarajan, V. 2016. *The Three Box Solution: A Strategy for Leading Innovation.* Boston: Harvard Business Review Press.

Institute of Medicine (IOM). 2007. *Preventing Medication Errors.* Washington, DC: National Academies Press.

———. 2006. "Medication Errors Injure 1.5 Million People and Cost Billions of Dollars Annually." Published July 20. www8.nationalacademies.org/onpinews/newsitem.aspx?RecordD=11623.

———. 2000. *To Err Is Human: Building a Safer Health System.* Washington, DC: National Academies Press.

Joshi, M. S., E. R. Ransom, D. B. Nash, and S. B. Ransom. 2014. *The Healthcare Quality Book: Vision, Strategy, and Tools.* Chicago: Health Administration Press.

Kotter, J. P. 2014. *Accelerate: Building Strategic Agility for a Faster-Moving World.* Boston: Harvard Business Review Press.

———. 2012. *Leading Change.* Boston: Harvard Business Review Press.

Kouzes, J. M., and B. Z. Posner. 2003. *The Leadership Challenge,* 3rd ed. San Francisco: Jossey-Bass.

Samit, J. 2015. *Disrupt You: Master Personal Transformation, Seize Opportunity, and Thrive in the Era of Endless Innovation.* New York: Flatiron.

Schimpff, S. C. 2012. *The Future of Health Care Delivery: Why It Must Change and How It Will Affect You.* Washington, DC: Potomac.

Spear, S. J. 2009. *The High-Velocity Edge: How Market Leaders Leverage Operational Excellence to Beat the Competition.* New York: McGraw-Hill.

Tett, G. 2015. *The Silo Effect: The Peril of Expertise and the Promise of Breaking Down Barriers.* New York: Simon & Schuster.

Topol, E. 2015. *The Patient Will See You Now: The Future of Medicine Is in Your Hands.* New York: Basic.

Wennberg, J. E. 2010. *Tracking Medicine: A Researcher's Quest to Understand Health Care.* New York: Oxford University Press.

White, K. R., and J. R. Griffith. 2016. *The Well-Managed Healthcare Organization,* 8th ed. Chicago: Health Administration Press.

# THE EVOLUTION OF LEADERSHIP IN HEALTHCARE

Bernard J. Healey

## Learning Objectives

After completing this chapter, the reader should be able to

- describe the most important leadership styles for healthcare organizations,
- discuss the major differences between transactional leadership and transformational leadership,
- understand the importance of communication skills in the success of the leadership style adopted, and
- discuss the value of leadership styles in rebuilding healthcare organizations.

## Key Terms and Concepts

- Contingency theory
- Creative destruction
- Empowerment
- Least-preferred coworker (LPC) scale
- Scientific management
- Servant leadership
- 10X companies

## Introduction

In his book titled *A Team of Teams: New Rules of Engagement for a Complex World*, retired Gen. Stanley McChrystal (2015) discussses the process he followed in restructuring the management style of the Joint Special Operations Command in 2004. McChrystal saw a need to change from a rigid command structure to a cooperative team approach because the command faced a new type of enemy in Iraqi insurgents that had adopted a different strategy of waging war than US forces had encountered in the past.

McChrystal then compared the efficiency level of the US military with the tenets of **scientific management**, discovered and made famous by efficiency expert and management guru Frederick Winslow Taylor in the early 1900s. Taylor's theory of scientific management was widely accepted as the best way to organize production because it emphasizes one right way to perform every aspect of a job, resulting in efficient production, reduced waste, and increased profit for the organization.

Scientific management theory became so popular that almost every organization evolved into a bureaucracy where management ruled and the worker became expendable. In fact, Taylor is said to have stated that managers did the thinking while the workers did only what they were told to do by the managers. Modern military management, too, evolved along scientific management theory lines. In his assessment, McChrystal (2015) determined that US military failures in Iraq resulted directly from inadequate war management techniques that could not work in a changing environment manipulated by a very different enemy.

This same revelation has occurred in many successful healthcare organizations over the past four decades. As we see more and more **creative destruction** and disruptive innovation taking place throughout the US economy, businesses—including in the healthcare industry—are moving from management to leadership as the answer to capturing or reviving their fortunes.

In the case of healthcare, the first step is to tear down its bureaucratic organizational structure and unlearn the scientific management style of operating. This unlearning is easier said than done because it has been such a large part, for such a long time, of how healthcare organizations are run. As McChrystal discovered, the US healthcare system must rid itself of its outdated structure and management techniques before it can become comfortable with a decentralized structure run by leaders. We will always need managers in healthcare organizations, but the value of leadership must be unleashed as well to respond to the new realities of the healthcare delivery workplace.

**Scientific management**
The theory of studying work processes to increase productivity.

**Creative destruction**
The use of capital resources to devise a product or service that is more valuable than the original capital.

## Movement from Bureaucracy and Scientific Management to Leadership

Both leaders and managers have been known to use leadership skills in the workplace, but the success of scientific management could not be ignored in the United States because it increased productivity and resulted in growing profits for businesses.

Leaders are traditionally called into service during periods of conflict, to which they bring special qualities that allow them to influence others, thereby improving the chances of success in resolving the conflict. This section discusses some studies and leadership research conducted to discover and describe specific behaviors or styles that have emerged over time, with an emphasis on those of effective leaders. Although not an exhaustive review of the leadership literature, the discussion points out important leadership styles that can be appropriate for use in healthcare organizations.

### Research on Leadership Style

In recent years, interest has increased in documenting the behaviors exhibited by successful leaders, perhaps as a result of the difficulties experienced by bureaucracies and managers trying to survive environmental change. While numerous studies support a movement to decentralize organizational structures that features more leadership and less management—which allows organizations to adapt rather than follow a prescribed plan—leadership styles over time warrant an extended discussion as well.

The first research projects related to leadership behaviors and styles began around 1930, with the most important research into leadership being conducted in the past 60 years. We start with a discussion of what leadership style means today, with some examples from industry to help set the stage. Later, we turn to early research in the academic arena and in the field of business. Last, discussion turns to insights about leadership style and behaviors in the tumultuous healthcare industry.

### What Leadership Style Means Today

To gain an understanding of leaders' styles, we first consider a research study by Jim Collins and Morten T. Hansen (2011), reported in their book *Great by Choice*. Collins and Hansen determined that some companies thrive on chaos while others do not, and they attempted to find out why. They labeled those that thrive in chaotic circumstances **10X companies** because the so-called winners in their study overperformed their respective industry indexes by at least 10 times.

**10X companies** Business entities that have achieved superior growth over time, by a factor of ten over their counterparts.

One example of a 10X company is Southwest Airlines. From 1972 to 2002, the company experienced seemingly every possible chaotic disruption and continued to deliver a superior service while satisfying all of its stakeholders. A key element of that success was Southwest's leader—and his leadership style—over that 30-year period.

Herb Kelleher is a founder of Southwest Airlines and served as its executive chairman from 1978 to 2008. The airline has been profitable for almost 40 years, and Kelleher grew the business in the face of a hostile environment during every year of his tenure. His leadership style was effective in terms of every available measurement index, including relationships with the external environment of suppliers and news media. According to Collins and Hansen (2011), Southwest is an example of a 10X company by virtue of its average 25 percent rate of return per year over a 30-year period, from $10,000 invested in 1972 to $200,000 in 2002. Despite oil embargoes, union disputes, intense competition, and a limited number of available passengers, Kelleher accomplished this growth because he understood early in his leadership career the relationship between happy, passionate employees and superb customer service. He succeeded in building a fun-loving workplace culture that made people—employees and customers—want to experience Southwest Airlines. This transformational leader (transformational leadership is discussed in more detail later in the chapter) kept costs and waste low and improved quality through the collective action he and his beloved staff undertook.

### *Early Academic Leadership Research*

Much of the early leadership research was funded by grants to colleges and universities to learn about the value of leadership, especially in business organizations. That research tended to focus on leadership traits and leadership styles or behaviors because these variables could be discovered through questionnaires, which were easily converted into publishable research articles. Because definitions of leadership vary and consensus is still lacking on the best approach (trait versus style) to leadership research, this text covers a few select studies of the styles and behaviors of leaders that fit healthcare organizations.

### Lewin's Leadership Styles

Kurt Lewin, a psychologist, offered a strong foundation in the 1930s for the discussion of leaders' behavior to come later. His research uncovered three major styles of leadership:

- Autocratic
- Democratic
- Laissez-faire

The autocratic style entails all power being kept by the leader in forcing his or her will on the followers, sometimes through rewards but mostly by frightening followers with potential punishments. The democratic leader shares his or her power equally with followers. The leader who uses a laissez-faire style gives virtually all power to the followers—and by granting that power relinquishes any responsibility for organizational success or failure.

One of Lewin's early studies was conducted at the University of Iowa. It concentrated on characterizing two of the aforementioned leadership styles, autocratic and democratic (Lussier and Achua 2010). The autocratic style involves the leader making all decisions and telling the lower-level employees what to do and how to do it (Lewin, Lippit, and White 1939). This leadership style may be seen as similar to a manager using organizational power to get the work done. It is an excellent style to bring into a discussion about leadership in healthcare facilities because many of these organizations still struggle to preserve the power of the executive suite.

Further along the continuum of leadership styles is the democratic style of leadership. Leaders practicing democratic leadership are much more likely than autocratic leaders to advocate for participatory decision making. The followers are requested by the leader to share with her their thoughts regarding impending decisions.

According to Lussier and Achua (2010), a second major research study by Lewin, completed at The Ohio State University in the 1950s, used a comprehensive questionnaire to discover whether two variables—consideration and initiating structure—can determine the focus of leadership style and behaviors. A consideration orientation was defined as the leader offering emotional support, friendliness, and general work-related support to followers. Leading with an initiating structure approach was defined as assigning tasks, clarifying expectations, and defining how work should be done. As can be seen, this study was similar to Lewin's University of Iowa research, the main difference being the wording of the two variables studied. Dubrin (2016) points out that this study largely influenced future research that tested leaders' behavior, attitudes, and styles.

## Likert's Human Relations Research

Lussier and Achua's (2010) work discusses another academic study of leadership, this one conducted at the University of Michigan under principal investigator Rensis Likert. This study examined the types of leadership that increased worker productivity and job satisfaction. Again, two factors were considered: an employee orientation and a production orientation. Likert and his colleagues defined the employee orientation in leadership as a human relations style, in which the leader pays attention to his followers' personal needs. The production orientation considered only the technical aspects of the work, concentrating on how the work was accomplished. Likert and colleagues found that leaders with an employee orientation were more concerned about their followers and their personal growth. Leaders exhibiting the production orientation focused on the task to be accomplished and demonstrated few if any human relations–style behaviors. The conclusion offered by Likert and colleagues supported a finding that an employee orientation usually resulted in better outcomes than did the production orientation (Lussier and Achua 2010).

### Path–Goal Theory

The path–goal theory was developed in 1971 by psychologist Robert House (1971). It factors into leadership style two separate pieces of work concerning motivation: goal setting and expectancy theory. Path–goal theory is concerned with the level of worker motivation required to achieve organizational goals. The motivating force set forth by the organization depends on the value of the goals to the worker and whether the worker believes she can achieve the goals.

According to path–goal theory, the leader's major responsibilities include clarifying what needs to be done, removing roadblocks to goal accomplishment, and increasing the opportunity for follower satisfaction at work (House 1971). In the context of the theories discussed earlier, path–goal theory may be seen as incorporating multiple styles of leadership with the major goals of increasing worker productivity while keeping the morale of followers high. It is among the first leadership theories to account for employees' concerns as they attempt to reach their assigned goals, such as limited resources or management interference. In the framework of this theory, the leader is expected to work on employees' behalf to ensure that they have what they need to meet the goals.

House (1971) proposed that leaders may use one of four leadership styles to achieve success: supportive leadership, directive leadership, participative leadership, or achievement-oriented leadership. The style of leadership used depends primarily on the group characteristics and the task being performed.

If we were to apply House's path–goal theory to today's changing healthcare environment, we would likely conclude that his participative leadership style works best.

The path–goal theory of leadership emphasizes the importance of effectiveness for healthcare organization operations. It also alerts the leader to numerous leadership styles that can be mixed and matched depending on the group to be led and the task being undertaken. In addition, it is a valuable model for thinking about leadership because path–goal theory aids in understanding the importance of matching the leader's style with the situation. For example, the approach to providing leadership in a modern operating room or emergency department differs greatly from providing leadership today in most other departments in a hospital.

Although this is a complicated theory, it is worth consideration because it supports the prevailing recommendations for empowering employees when they are prepared for the responsibility. Dubrin (2016) details a number of suggestions for leaders to influence the performance of followers on the basis of path–goal theory:

- The leader may help the worker by coaching him or her and providing direction on ways to achieve the most important goals.
- The leader may help the worker clarify expectations.
- The leader may work to eliminate barriers to goal achievement.
- The leader may recognize employees who have been successful in goal achievement.

### Fiedler's Contingency Theory

Fred Fiedler (1967) developed the **contingency theory** of leadership, which essentially posits that no single best way exists to structure an organization. Contingency theory helps decision makers factor in the situation at hand when selecting a leader, and it aids leaders in determining which leadership style or behavior to use. This theory also is based on two factors for analysis: relationship-motivated factors and task-motivated factors. Contingency theory includes three important situational variables that can affect the success or failure of a leader:

- Leader–member relations
- Task structure
- Position power

Bolden and colleagues (2011) interpret contingency theory to mean that managers who take a task-oriented approach perform better than those with a relationship orientation in situations that already have in place good leader–member relations, structured tasks, and either weak or strong position power. Dubrin (2016) points out that leadership results in the best outcomes when the leader is placed in a situation that closely matches her style.

To determine a leader's style in the contingency theory framework, the **least-preferred coworker (LPC) scale** may be used. A questionnaire developed by Fiedler and Chemers (1984) asks the leader to think about the person she least enjoys working with. The leader is then asked to identify how she feels about this person. The questionnaire is designed to produce a score that separates task-oriented leaders from relationship-oriented leaders. Individuals who score low on the LPC scale are effective at completing tasks; high-scoring LPC leaders are more relationship oriented.

### Servant Leadership

The concept of **servant leadership**, introduced by Robert Greenleaf in 1970 with his famous essay titled "The Servant as Leader," has gained a large

---

**Contingency theory**
Theory that states there is no best way to organize an organization.

**Least-preferred coworker (LPC) scale**
Theory that considers the concept of a fellow employee with whom others prefer not to work on a project.

**Servant leadership**
Style of leadership that occurs when serving and leading are in harmony.

following in a variety of settings, including religious, community, and not-for-profit, because it can be used by individuals who are not in a formal position of leadership (Greenleaf 1996). According to Autry (2001), the most important function of leaders is to demonstrate their usefulness as a resource for their followers. Bolden and colleagues (2011) note that servant leaders follow the leadership path out of a desire to serve others rather than to lead followers.

Also known as informal or quiet leadership, this leadership style usually features a leader who values the opinions of others to the point where he involves followers in decision making and is concerned about their personal growth and quality of work life at the organization. The servant leader has a strong motivational impact on others by demonstrating his integrity and generosity. Servant leaders can also gain power over others by exhibiting their values and high ideals.

Maxwell (2007) discusses the servant leadership style of Dan Cathy, president of Chick-fil-A. Although it is smaller than competitors such as McDonald's, Cathy argues that his company will beat the competition, not through size but through service to others. His leadership style was demonstrated through one of his leadership tools, a nine-inch, 100 percent horsehair shoe brush. He used the shoe brush to shine Maxwell's shoes during an interview for a leadership book. Cathy is known for such acts of service to customers and employees, exhibiting his sense of humility despite his great wealth and power.

## Inspired Leadership

An inspiring leader has the ability to instill optimism and hope in all of his or her employees. Such leaders are always optimistic about the future of the organization and its most important resource, its people. Inspired leadership also has been associated with responsibility on the job, enthusiasm for the company, and resilience in responding to setbacks. In the US healthcare system's attempt to redesign care delivery, all these qualities are important and even required.

Businesses today value inspired leadership because of its aim to motivate followers to the achievement of lofty goals. According to Zenger, Folkman, and Edinger (2009), the ability of the leader to inspire his followers usually results in increased levels of commitment, satisfaction, and retention. These results represent important accomplishments for businesses, such as healthcare, that deliver services through highly trained professionals.

Healthcare employees who do not practice good corporate citizenship and are constantly looking for new employment can trigger serious consequences in both the short term and long term for the healthcare facility. Good corporate citizenship means speaking highly of both the organization and its leaders even when away from the workplace. It is a sign of employees' happiness at work and can speak volumes to potential future employees and customers of the organization they represent. Successful organizations constantly seek new talent to replace retiring workers and current employees who do not fit well with the culture of the organization, and a culture of good corporate citizenship enlarges the potential employee pool.

Zenger, Folkman, and Edinger (2009) further note that because the leader typically plays a crucial role in the improvement of productivity in an organization, leading with inspiration is a key factor in building confidence among employees while empowering them in the belief that their capabilities are sufficient to try new procedures or processes and successfully implement new ideas.

Inspirational leaders also develop trust and ultimately become role models for all of the people they come in contact with every day. In fact, the most effective leaders are also excellent role models for their organization and followers (Zenger, Folkman, and Edinger 2009). Horsager (2009) points to numerous studies that strongly support the notion that trust is built over time because followers are continually watching what the leader says and how the leader acts. Leaders must learn that when they demonstrate authenticity, they allow their employees to trust them to meet the challenges faced together as healthcare delivery is reinvented.

## Transactional Leadership

Transaction-style leadership involves an agreement between the leader and followers as to how they will meet the organizational goals. The agreement calls for a transaction whereby the followers agree to listen to the leader in return for some payment for their effort. Lussier and Achua (2016) suggest that the transactional style of leadership rewards followers for specific behaviors that benefit the organization. This style can also inflict punishment in return for the followers practicing the wrong behaviors. This leadership style, frequently seen in bureaucratic organizations, relies on the use of organizational, legitimate, reward, and coercive power.

Although transactional style leaders typically do not move into the realm of true leadership, they tend to use compassionate management skills. That said, they are obsessed with efficient production through the use of standard routines and procedures and by basing rewards and punishments on whether staff follow the leader's direction.

The transactional style of leadership follows many of the recommendations of the scientific management school of thought. One of its limitations is that little thought is given to shifting to a new plan if the environment changes during the original plan's execution.

Transactional leadership focuses on organizational rules and regulations; its leaders look for short-term achievements rather than the long-term growth of the organization and its people. According to Podsakoff, Podsakoff, and Kuskova (2010), people who practice transactional leadership are more interested in the daily routines of leaders and followers than in expressing concern for the future of the organization and its employees. These leaders also show little if any concern for employee creativity and consider followers to lack self-motivation.

This style is also known as management by exception. It places a major focus on supervision, organization, and group performance whereby the leader acts more as a coach than a leader. The emphasis on short-term rewards and punishments on the basis of performance renders transactional leadership ineffective in a vision for the future and using change management to attain that vision.

This style works well in the handling of a short-term crisis where a rapid response is required and secondary effects of actions are not a concern. In everyday situations, the transactional leader works to sustain the current culture of the organization and is passive in the face of any attempt to change it. The entire emphasis of this leader is on the standardization of practices to be efficient and increase worker productivity.

Observers tend to underestimate the negative impact transactional leadership behaviors have on leaders' effectiveness. The use of contingent reward and punishment characteristic of this style has been linked to an inability to establish credibility, gain trust with employees, and elicit superior performance from staff (Podsakoff, Podsakoff, and Kuskova 2010).

## Transformational Leadership

The transformational style of leadership is characterized by humanism and concern for followers, similar to the types of behaviors found in informal leaders (Miner 2013). As with informal leadership, transformational leaders' concern for followers is an important prerequisite for gaining the trust of individuals, which is a primary factor in facilitating the change process.

Transformational leadership is composed of four behavioral dimensions: idealized influence, inspirational motivation, individual consideration, and intellectual stimulation (Lussier and Achua 2016). The situation faced by the leader determines which behavioral dimension is appropriate for success in ensuring that change occurs.

Transformational leaders have the ability to move large groups of individuals beyond their self-interest toward the fulfillment of the greater good of the organization (Dubrin 2016). This effort becomes much easier for the leaders and followers if the organization has reached consensus on its purpose or mission.

The transformational leader is concerned about his staff and their personal development. He may use a charismatic approach (discussed in more detail later) to convince followers that he has the right vision for the company. Dubrin (2016) suggests that this vision must include values capable of motivating the followers to want to be part of the organization after the leader's transformation takes place. By including this appealing vision with the opportunity for the personal growth of the follower, the leader can gain total buy-in by the followers. The followers trust this leader and will follow with a belief that the leader is heading in the right direction to achieve organizational goals.

The transformational style can thus be equated to an exceptional form of influence over followers that allows them to achieve extraordinary accomplishments. The transformational leader spends a great deal of time building strong, positive relationships with most people in the organization to influence it in a positive direction. This relationship between leader and followers becomes so strong that followers do what they are requested to do because of their respect for the leader. This is a key requirement for the leader to successfully change the way the organization has done business for a long time.

In healthcare delivery, the transformational leader also works to help followers understand the need for change. In some respects, she is asking followers to unlearn behaviors they have practiced for years. Transformational leaders understand that most followers know when quality is poor and costs are high. The difficulty is in convincing followers to implement change *now*.

Here is a key juncture where the concept of trust arises in the leader–follower relationship. Lussier and Achua (2016) point out that followers must believe strongly in the integrity of the transformational leader to place themselves at risk to follow her dream or vision, and to do so at a moment's notice. Stevenson and Kaafarani (2011) note that transformational leaders are persistent, committed, and unafraid of failure. These qualities help them succeed at building teams that are exceptional innovators. Leadership and innovation is discussed in more detail in chapter 4.

### Charismatic Leadership

Charisma has been mentioned already in this chapter because of its importance in the personal power held by a leader. In its simplest form, charisma is an appealing set of characteristics of an individual that influences others to be in that individual's company. It may be described as a charming personality that captivates listeners when this gifted individual speaks.

The charismatic nature of leadership has always been part of the researcher's interest when testing the successes and failures of leaders in a multitude of situations. According to Bolden and colleagues (2011), the charismatic leader becomes a solid role model for the values of importance to his organization. This modeling allows the leader to hold a compelling level of authority over followers primarily due to the inspirational qualities he exhibits. This effect usually manifests in increased productivity and improved satisfaction with employment by the followers of a charismatic leader.

Antonakis, Fenley, and Liechti (2012) suggest that while many people believe one is born with charisma, it is actually a skill that can be learned, though it requires a great deal of practice. The authors argue that many so-called charismatic leadership tactics (CLTs), if learned, can improve one's ability to influence others. Teaching the reader how to be charismatic is outside the scope of this text. Suffice to say that CLTs can be acquired and an individual can gain a measure of personal power through the development of charismatic qualities.

That said, whether you aspire to be a charismatic leader or consider yourself to be one already, chances are you will encounter at least one charismatic leader in your career. The rest of this section discusses the implications of charismatic leadership for healthcare.

One of the most important aspects of a charismatic leader is the ability to communicate a vision of the future that can excite followers into action designed to make the vision reality. This message of a reachable future can be a source of motivation for all staff, as the excitement produced allows complete follower engagement to occur in enacting the mission of the organization.

The US healthcare system depends on organizations capable of offering the best care possible with available resources. Built into this vision is the elimination of waste, elimination of "never events," improved interaction with patients, and improved health outcomes by virtue of seeking care at the facility. This challenge is formidable for healthcare organizations because, as noted earlier, it requires most followers, especially physicians, to unlearn behaviors that have been practiced for a long period.

Jennings (2015) discovered that if a large number of employees distrust the business and the leaders of that business, employees likely will ignore the call for change coming forth from these leaders. This phenomenon places a new healthcare leader at a major disadvantage, considering all the changes she must make. More discussion on trust, its importance, and how to gain the trust needed to change one's organization is offered later in the book.

The power that comes from charisma can be utilized by so-called bad leaders as well as good leaders. A classic example of this leadership style in the hands of a bad leader is Adolph Hitler, who used his power to control large numbers of people and was the major figure responsible for hostilities leading to World War II. More recent examples include the use of charismatic power by bad leaders to amass wealth by using unethical or illegal tactics, often taking organizations into bankruptcy.

# The Concept of Best Leadership Practices

What style is best for leading a service-producing organization? Does one best style of leadership apply in the majority of US healthcare organizations? Many organizations have been plagued by failed attempts to adopt a comprehensive leadership approach in the past few decades. Coleman (2000) identified six leadership styles typically assumed by organizations, concluding that successful leaders do not rely on one style but rather use multiple styles in a given period.

Kotter (1999) notes that both management and leadership attributes are necessary for success in an increasingly complex business environment. He argues that organizations today are overmanaged and underled. Assuming this is an accurate assessment, what should be the compromise or balance between management and leadership in the delivery of healthcare services in this volatile environment? Healthcare leaders must spend more time setting the direction for the organization and give managers the responsibility to plan operations and budgets. This notion takes us back to our concept of providing the best care possible as the overriding organizational goal.

Latham (2014) argues that determining the measure of success—what constitutes "successful leadership" and the style that most reliably works in attaining that success—is difficult. One common approach he cites is to hold out one measure of success, such as economic profit, and then claim that the leader was successful using a given style. When the organization's overall success is dissected and examined, however, numerous problems with that claim are evident, as Latham shows.

Ultimately, no theory of leadership offers a complete answer to the multitude of challenges faced by healthcare organizations in the twenty-first century. Instead, what has become clear is that the effectiveness of leadership depends on the fit between the leader, his style, and the situation in which the leader is placed. A leadership style that has been effective with one group in one situation may not work with all groups in all situations. Therefore, wise healthcare leaders have realized they must have a general knowledge and grasp of several leadership styles and use the one that works best in a given situation. In fact, the best leaders may use several leadership styles at the same time. The earlier example of Kelleher's leadership ability most likely involved transformational leadership and servant leadership combined, with a focus on the personal growth of his employees and offering superb service to the customers.

This understanding of leadership style adaptability underscores Latham's (2014) argument that little agreement has been reached among observers on which style of leadership works best. The unfortunate result of that lack of consensus is that, even when poor results are reported, few theories of leadership are dropped from use.

One of the most important effects of successful, strong leadership is in the culture of innovation that emerges. Stevenson and Kaafarani (2011) conclude that healthcare organizations and their top leadership team must become focused on innovation to deliver profitable growth while eliminating waste and improving the quality of all services delivered to a now highly informed consumer. The catalyst for a change in the healthcare delivery model must be innovative leadership that, if executed appropriately, eliminates the confusion currently seen among many who work in healthcare. This level of leadership can be effective in convincing people that they can, in fact, accomplish goals they previously believed were impossible.

A final leadership lesson learned from McChrystal (2015) relates to understanding the difference between efficiency and adaptability in successful team leadership. In the days when scientific management worked well in a stable environment, efficiency and effectiveness were essentially the same concept. Companies could make solid plans with the assurance that rapid change in the environment was not likely or even possible. Now, change is unleashed constantly by the nature of a macroeconomic environment and through shifts specific to healthcare, such as new reimbursement techniques. These changes make predictions of the future difficult, if not impossible.

Rather than following a path that had ensured the successes of the past, McChrystal (2015) advocates for developing the ability to adapt to rapidly changing circumstances. Noting that attempts to merely block change—typically seen in top-down organizations with strict rules of management—are doomed to fail in a rapidly changing business environment, McChrystal writes that the resilient, or adaptable, organization can make changes rapidly, where the efficient organization cannot. The staff of resilient organizations have **empowerment** to act immediately without approval by using common sense to respond to the changes they face. This is a good lesson for healthcare organizations to learn as they go about changing the design of the organization and training their leaders for an unknown future.

**Empowerment**
The freedom conferred by management on lower-level employees to make decisions without asking for permission.

## Summary

In recent years, the study of leadership has become popular in part to address the turmoil caused by globalization, disruptive innovation, technology, and intense competition from nontraditional sources. This threatening environment has forced a large number of businesses to change their bureaucratic organizational structure to a more organic one headed by leaders rather than managers. This need for change has been felt in the US healthcare delivery system as well.

Many styles or behaviors of leaders should be considered as healthcare delivery moves from bureaucracy to a decentralized structure. These styles of leadership have been identified by research projects looking at different variables that seem to affect one's ability to lead followers. Among the important leadership models are contingency theory, path–goal theory, servant leadership, inspired leadership, transactional leadership, and transformational leadership. The overriding themes of the majority of studies include concern for people versus concern for production or task. The implication of all this research seems to be that successful leadership typically depends on the particular leader, followers, and situation in which the leader is placed.

## Discussion Questions

1. Explain the role of leadership style in effective leadership.
2. Which leadership style or behavior is best suited for healthcare organizations? Why?
3. Name and explain the major differences between transactional leadership and transformational leadership.
4. Explain the advantages and disadvantages of charismatic leadership.

## References

Antonakis, J., M. Fenley, and S. Liechti. 2012. "Learning Charisma: Transform Yourself into the Person Others Want to Follow." *Harvard Business Review* 90 (6): 127–30.

Autry, J. A. 2001. *The Servant Leader: How to Build a Creative Team, Develop Great Morale, and Improve Bottom-Line Performance.* New York: Three Rivers Press.

Bolden, R., B. Hawkins, J. Gosling, and S. Taylor. 2011. *Exploring Leadership: Individual, Organizational & Societal Perspectives.* New York: Oxford University Press.

Coleman, D. 2000. "Leadership That Gets Results." *Harvard Business Review* 78 (2): 78–90.

Collins, J., and M. T. Hansen. 2011. *Great by Choice.* New York: Harper Collins.

Dubrin, A. J. 2016. *Leadership: Research Findings, Practice, and Skills,* 8th ed. Boston: Cengage Learning.

Fiedler. F. E. 1967. *A Theory of Leadership Effectiveness.* New York: McGraw-Hill.

Fiedler, F. M., and M. M. Chemers. 1984. *Improving Leadership Effectiveness: The Leader Match Concept.* New York: Wiley.

Greenleaf, R. K. 1996. *On Becoming a Servant Leader: The Private Writings of Robert K Greenleaf,* edited by D. M. Frick and L. C. Spears. San Francisco: Jossey-Bass.

Horsager, D. 2009. *The Trust Edge: How Top Leaders Gain Faster Results, Deeper Relationships, and a Stronger Bottom Line.* New York: Free Press.

House, R. J. 1971. "A Path-Goal Theory of Leader Effectiveness." *Administrative Science Quarterly* 16: 321–28.

Jennings, J. 2015. *Creating Urgency and Growth: The High-Speed Company.* New York: Penguin.

Kotter, J. P. 1999. *What Leaders Really Do.* Boston: Harvard Business School Press.

Latham, J. R. 2014. "Leadership for Quality and Innovation: Challenges, Theories, and a Framework for Future Research." *Quality Management Journal* 21 (1): 11–15.

Lewin, K., R. Lippit, and R. K. White. 1939. "Patterns of Aggressive Behavior in Experimentally Created Social Climate." *Journal of Social Psychology* 10: 271–301.

Lussier, R. N., and C. F. Achua. 2016. *Leadership: Theory, Application and Skill Development,* 6th ed. Boston: Cengage Learning.

———. 2010. *Leadership Theory Application and Skill Development,* 4th ed. Mason, OH: South Western.

Maxwell, J. C. 2007. *The 21 Irrefutable Laws of Leadership: Follow Them and People Will Follow You.* Nashville, TN: Thomas Nelson.

McChrystal, S. 2015. *A Team of Teams: New Rules of Engagement for a Complex World.* New York: Penguin.

Miner, R. C. 2013. "Informal Leaders." *Journal of Leadership, Accountability and Ethics* 10 (4): 57–61.

Podsakoff, N. P., P. M. Podsakoff, and V. V. Kuskova. 2010. "Dispelling Misconceptions and Providing Guidelines for Leader Reward and Punishment Behavior." *Science Direct* 53: 291–303.

Stevenson, J., and B. Kaafarani. 2011. *Breaking Away: How Great Leaders Create Innovation That Drives Sustainable Growth and Why Others Fail.* New York: McGraw-Hill.

Zenger, J. H., J. R. Folkman, and S. K. Edinger. 2009. *The Inspiring Leader: Unlocking the Secrets of How Extraordinary Leaders Motivate.* New York: McGraw-Hill.

# LEADERSHIP SKILLS

# LEADERSHIP THEORY

Bernard J. Healey

## Learning Objectives

After completing this chapter, the reader should be able to

- understand the theoretical models related to leadership development,
- realize the importance of organizational purpose in leadership development,
- understand how power develops in an organization, and
- understand the value of developing personal power to improve leadership abilities.

## Key Terms and Concepts

- Bureaucratic organization
- Charisma
- Conflict management
- Culture
- Disruptive innovation
- Leadership development

- Organizational structure
- Paradigm
- Power base
- Sources of power
- Turbulence

## Introduction

The need for leadership in organizations is a relatively new concept that has only gained importance in recent decades. In fact, as mentioned earlier, much of the research regarding leadership theory has been conducted just during the past 60 years. Prior to that time, most organizations were structured as bureaucracies and run by managers (in the literal sense, as described in an earlier chapter), and little appreciation for the topic of leadership was evident. This is not to say that leaders did not exist throughout US history. The point is that the role of leaders in US business was largely misunderstood. The principles of management seemed to work well in most businesses based in the United States, so leadership was rarely given serious attention.

Leadership is a difficult topic to both explain and understand. The major reason for this difficulty is the continual and frequent emergence of new information and theory about what constitutes leadership. The theoretical base concerning leadership has always been considered a work in progress. In recent years, this topic has become an important concern for companies struggling with intense competition and threats to their survival, whether they are for-profit or not-for-profit businesses.

In addition, a great deal of recent interest has been noted in determining the differences between managers and leaders and the value of training managers in the principles of leadership. Leaders should be able to inspire confidence in their followers to complete organizational tasks over time. Leadership represents one of those intangible concepts that can be sensed in the short run but measured only through organizational results in the long term.

**Conflict management**
The concept that discord or disagreement can be helpful for growth but needs to be managed.

College-level management textbooks historically contained only one brief chapter on leadership, if they covered leadership at all. Even less space was allocated to organizational culture, though the importance of culture has long been discussed in management meetings. Conflict and **conflict management** were absent from discussions about the management of organizations because the bureaucratic structure does not support conflict and attempts to block conflict from ever occurring through rules and regulations. Finally, the topics of creativity and innovation have largely been absent from management literature and discussions. They simply were considered unimportant to the operation of a **bureaucratic organization** because change was traditionally blocked.

**Bureaucratic organization**
A corporate structure that focuses on rules and regulations to achieve efficiency.

In recent years, this lack of interest in leadership has seen a reversal, as change—**disruptive innovation** in particular—emerged in the headlines of major newspapers, reflecting the change phenomenon occurring throughout US business and industry. Dobbs, Manyika, and Woetzel (2015) point out that most company executives who had never thought about being disrupted by competitors are now expecting disruption and becoming concerned about the severity of the disruption. They are slowly realizing that the only way to prepare for disruption in their business is through enlightened leadership and empowered followers. Some proactive businesses have chosen leadership development as the key to becoming the disrupters rather than the disrupted business. In other words, rather than blocking change, they now actively seek to exploit change. As a result, the need to incorporate leadership in organizational structure has achieved great importance as more and more companies throughout the United States become disrupted and, in many cases, disappear from existence.

**Disruptive innovation**
A new way of operating that typically begins in smaller companies and diffuses throughout an industry, causing upheaval to other businesses in that industry.

In his book *Confronting Capitalism: Real Solutions for a Troubled Economic System,* Kotler (2015) discusses turbulence as the new normal in the business environment. He defines **turbulence** as a state of unpredictability that causes rapid changes in the organization's environment. When we see chaos in our business environment, we tend to think that it is temporary and will soon return to normal. In fact, this chaotic environment may be the new normal, which requires a change in **organizational structure** to address it. For successful companies, this new structure likely entails an organic, decentralized framework requiring new operating techniques.

Naturally, the decline of the bureaucratic organizational structure, along with unrelenting competitive forces and the explosion of new technology, has caused management to lose most of its influence on the way companies work. Managers will always be needed to ensure organizational control, but the principles of management no longer work well in our ever-changing, technology-driven workplace. A decentralized organizational structure run by self-managed work teams, while difficult to manage, thrives under leadership that supports employee empowerment.

All of these factors make **leadership development** a virtual mandate for a new type of employee in a reinvented workplace. This expectation is especially valid for healthcare organizations struggling with boosting productivity to reduce healthcare costs while improving quality. This call to develop leadership becomes important not only for those in charge but also for the newly empowered employee. In fact, leadership development is emerging as a popular training exercise among most US companies. Such training programs should emphasize the following aspects of leadership:

- Culture building
- The change process
- Creativity and innovation
- Conflict management

At a glance, we see that leadership development includes some skills that are not typically found in management development programs.

A paradigm shift has been seen in the way success is perceived in the new world of rapid environmental change. A **paradigm** is a pattern or system of how activities are performed to ensure successful completion. The term *paradigm shift* became popular with Thomas Kuhn's (1962) model of scientific revolutions. According to Kuhn, science moves forward through revolutionary steps. For our purposes, a paradigm shift reflects a substantial change in the way healthcare services are produced and delivered to an increasingly knowledgeable consumer. Thaler (2015) suggests that paradigm shifts may

**Turbulence**
A state of chaotic occurrences causing unpredictable change.

**Organizational structure**
The way activities and positions are organized toward the accomplishment of goals.

**Leadership development**
A series of educational programs designed to facilitate the growth of leadership traits in individuals.

**Paradigm**
A pattern or system of how activities are performed to ensure successful completion.

take place following the occurrence of anomalies that cannot be adequately explained by the current paradigm or popular theory.

This type of paradigm shift has been seen in successful businesses in terms of the way they operate in the modern US economy. Here, bureaucracies have been replaced by decentralized organizational structures that require decentralized teams as well as leaders rather than controlling managers. The problem has been that many organizations, especially in healthcare, have not recognized the need for this change and have attempted to operate with the bureaucratic structure run by managers who may not have any leadership skills. The anomaly that has occurred is the failure of many of these previously successful organizations to question the relevance of the bureaucratic type of organizational structure. This trend is especially prevalent in organizations that are labor intensive and deliver services to people, such as healthcare.

Paradigm shifts have occurred previously in the healthcare industry over the past few decades, particularly in medicine. For example, for years scientists believed ulcers were caused by stress leading to excessive stomach acidity and that a medication called Tagamet was the appropriate treatment to reduce the acid. Then, Australian scientists Barry Marshall and Robin Warren claimed that ulcers are caused by a bacteria rather than excess acidity. To gain medical acceptance for this theory, Marshall went so far as to infect himself with the bacteria to develop an ulcer and treat himself with antibiotics (Hartford 2016). These scientists disrupted the healthcare industry, won a Nobel prize, and demonstrated the need for influence in order to lead.

In the current paradigm shift prevailing in healthcare, providers have encountered the types of disruptive change mentioned earlier and, in many cases, have begun to lose faith in traditional management techniques. As they come to grips with the fact that this rapidly changing environment is, in fact, the new normal, they look to leaders to help them deal with the unknown environment they face.

## A Brief History of Management and Managers

Managers have overseen activities since the beginning of business endeavors and the first attempts at commerce. Their skills increased in visibility as businesses grew and became complex organizations. Any time groups of individuals were threatened by a hostile external environment, the need for managers became even more evident. For centuries, large organizations placed managers in charge of their equally large bureaucracies, designed solely for efficiency. These managers made sure operations ran smoothly through the use of rules, regulations, rewards, and punishments. They used (and continue to use) organizational power, consisting of control through rewards and punishment, and legitimacy, because they were promoted by the organization to a management position. This type of bureaucratic organization worked well—until it stopped working well, because of the occurrence of constant, rapid change. In other words, bureaucratic organizations can function well for long periods as long as change in the environment is kept to a minimum. Organizations actively sought to maintain status quo by blocking change through rules and regulations.

The manager performed well because he had at his disposal several control mechanisms to improve efficiency and increase profits. Organizational conflict also was blocked through the sheer power of the manager. Communication consisted of managers talking to employees and employees listening if they chose to do so.

The enormous change experienced in the past few decades revealed the limitations of both bureaucracy and the management of people. At this point, successful organizations began to experiment with a new type of organizational structure characterized by a flattened hierarchy and the use of leaders rather than managers. Here, leadership began to gain prominence over management.

## The Shift to Leadership

Thousands of books and journal articles have been written about leadership, with a variety of definitions gaining popularity as more research of leaders and decentralized organizational structures was conducted. Common to these definitions is an essential characteristic: the ability to influence others. Wilkins and Carolin (2013) further point out that discussions about leadership almost always involve qualities that can inspire individuals and even nations to achieve above-average accomplishments. This power to motivate others is typically seen as a defining difference between leaders and managers.

Aside from these overarching aspects of leadership, however, Bolden and colleagues (2011) argue that a universally accepted definition of leadership is hard to find. They point to a lack of evidence that the appearance of leadership translates to improved organizational performance. Considering US business and industry invest so much time and money in leadership training, this finding is a compelling revelation.

One way to view this concern is to conclude that organizations spend a great deal of resources either training the wrong people for leadership or offering training programs that fail to provide relevant leadership training to the right people.

### Leadership Today

The many challenges facing the healthcare industry today are driving an overhaul in organizational structure, and particularly in the way organizations view and treat lower-level employees, to deal with these issues. Healthcare is being reformed: The patient has become a consumer, and third-party payers are becoming increasingly reluctant to pay for healthcare-related expenditures that fall outside of improved health outcomes. Thus, a change in the way healthcare is delivered is mandatory.

With that mandate, leadership development needs to be a priority for any healthcare facility that plans to remain relevant in the US healthcare delivery system.

## Leadership Theory

Before we begin to develop an explanation of leadership, we must develop a sound theoretical base for the concept of leadership. Theories usually represent an idea or a group of ideas used to explain a given event. Another way of looking at a theory is as an explanation of why things happen the way they do.

### The Value of Theory

A theory involves numerous concepts that are related and considered together that help us gain an enhanced understanding of a situation under investigation. To gain knowledge of a phenomenon, research data are gathered about the topic. Those charged with completing the research use the scientific method in an attempt to uncover the process involved in an occurrence and to make predictions concerning that occurrence. The more research that is completed on a given subject, the better is our collective understanding of that subject.

That said, though a great deal of research supporting the leadership concept is readily available, a large number of management theorists still believe that leadership is merely a small portion of a manager's daily duties. This belief is perpetuated by the many management textbooks that devote only one chapter to the concept of leadership and by the fact that a student may finish a college degree in management without ever taking a course in leadership.

Lussier and Achua (2016) argue that leadership theory needs to be developed to improve overall understanding of leaders and leadership, thereby providing a way to enhance leadership development. Leadership theory is useful in this endeavor because it offers a step-by-step approach to gaining knowledge of leaders' behavior and building an advanced theoretical model for leadership development. The reliability of such a model ultimately depends on the theory and all of the evidence gathered over time that supports the particular model.

## Building an Advanced Leadership Development Model

A large body of theoretical data support the notion that influence, power, purpose, and specific leadership skills are required for an individual to be an effective leader. These are the components that shape the concept of an advanced model of leadership. Exhibit 3.1 includes the foundations or building blocks of leadership, followed by further elevated skills of a leader. Once embedded, these components should lead to the achievement of both personal and organizational goals, which eventually merge to become similar. Such leaders can help organizations and institutions attain goals linked to operational imperatives, from deficit reduction in the federal government's budget to healthcare cost reduction and quality improvement in the US healthcare services delivery system.

To build a meaningful leadership development theoretical model, we must devise a classification of leadership theory divided into the following, eminently manageable, areas (Lussier and Achua 2016):

- Trait
- Behavioral
- Contingency
- Integrative

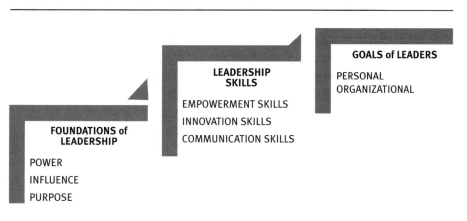

**GOALS of LEADERS**

PERSONAL
ORGANIZATIONAL

**LEADERSHIP SKILLS**

EMPOWERMENT SKILLS

INNOVATION SKILLS

COMMUNICATION SKILLS

**FOUNDATIONS of LEADERSHIP**

POWER

INFLUENCE

PURPOSE

**EXHIBIT 3.1**
Advanced Leadership Theory

Assigning manageable classifications such as these allows researchers to segment their research data into meaningful portions for additional research and theoretical development and to gain new meaning from their data.

Over the years, numerous leadership theories have been developed and, in many cases, rejected after intense follow-up research was conducted on the new theory. The best way to learn about leadership may be to look at past research to discover what works consistently in the real world. Reviewing research also offers one explanation of why new theories of leadership, seemingly reported on a daily basis, require testing to prove their validity.

To commence with building our advanced leadership development model, we focus on the components of leadership that have emerged as among the most common in effective leaders: power, influence, and purpose, ultimately leading to goal achievement.

## *Power*
### Development of Power

**Power base**
A foundation of authority, whether given by the organization or owned by the individual, that secures the right to lead.

Those studying the development of leadership tend to look first at how leaders develop their **power base**, which seems to be a prerequisite for becoming a leader. According to Bolden and colleagues (2011), leaders—whether formal or informal—possess the power to influence followers. In a bureaucratic organization, power usually results from an individual's location on the organizational chart. Those higher up on the chart are typically charged with developing the rules and regulations followed by individuals lower on the chart. This form of position power is a key aspect of leadership in a bureaucratic organization.

To influence individuals, one needs to have developed a base of power that can be drawn on when needed. This power must be acquired and then developed and used frequently. The research concerning power seems to indicate that the more power is used by an individual, the more powerful that individual usually becomes.

Fundamental questions to be answered in leadership theory development are (1) What is power? and (2) Why is power so important for leadership to emerge? Naim (2013) defines power as the unique ability to direct or prevent actions by individuals or groups of individuals using control or influence.

In a bureaucratic organization, the positional power referred to earlier belongs to the organization and, therefore, can never be owned by the current wielder of this power. In other words, if you are in a management position and leave the organization, this power remains with the organization and eventually is given to someone else. One reason many people never seek organizational power is that they recognize it may be a short-term situation that, once acquired, becomes difficult to leave behind.

## Sources and Types of Power

Lombardi and Schermerhorn (2007) discuss five **sources of power:**

- Rewards
- Punishment
- Legitimacy
- Expertise
- Referent

**Sources of power**
Rewards, punishment, legitimacy, expertise, and referent.

These power sources can be further classified as power that flows from the organization and power that is found in the individual.

As mentioned earlier, organizational power is given, and taken away, by the organization. Personal power, which consists of expertise (one of the aforementioned sources) and charisma, is owned, developed, and nurtured by the individual. This type of power can never be taken away because it is an inherent attribute of the individual rather than conferred by the organization. Of these two types of power, personal power is typically viewed as superior to organizational power, as upon leaving an organization, an individual's personal power leaves with her. It also tends to help alleviate fear in responding to change because the individual has confidence in her power base.

Individuals with advanced leadership skills recognize the limited value of organizational power, especially when attempting to make significant changes in the ways individuals and groups function. These leaders grasp the notion that change may hurt before it heals, placing them in a risky short-term environment, and they understand the value of developing their personal power before attempting to make large changes in an organization.

One does not have to be in a leadership position to have personal power. The ownership of this personal power in an organization can, in fact, make an individual a successful informal leader. This type of power is often found in entrepreneurs and is the main reason they tend to experience success in start-up businesses.

## How Leaders Gain Personal Power

Lussier and Achua (2016) point out that the personal power of the leader is acquired from the followers of the organization. The authors use the concept of referent power to explain the role of **charisma** in successful leadership activities. Referent power demonstrates the unique ability to appeal to the values and ideals of the followers, allowing the leader to offer inspirational messages. This charismatic nature, supplemented with a certain amount of expertise, motivates and influences employees to reach a high level or purpose in the organization. Because the individual has no fear of losing personal power, the leader may feel free to spend more time developing employees and

**Charisma**
The compelling attractiveness or charm of an individual that affords the individual personal power.

less time worrying about gaining favor with upper-level managers. In turn, employees have respect for a leader who is concerned about them and their personal growth, further bolstering the leader's personal power.

Much of a leader's personal power comes from the ability to both acquire charisma and demonstrate expertise. Individuals improve on these personal powers through training and practice. The most important revelation about acquiring personal power is that its traits belong to you, so you have reason to gain these abilities and keep them. They give you the power to lead any organization, especially service delivery organizations that rely so much on people.

### Leaders' Use of Personal Power

Considering that personal power is a critical ingredient of service delivery leadership, the development of this type of power is a primary necessity for the leaders of healthcare facilities facing reform. Charisma in particular is important in the use of communication skills to gain influence while explaining the purpose of the organization to employees. These communication skills are also critical in culture building and employee development.

To meet the vast majority of these challenges, the leader requires support from his followers, who need to be as committed as the leader is to problem solving. This collaboration among team members in turn requires leadership expertise and charisma from the leader. Problems become easier to solve when the leader and the team working on the solution share an understanding of the issue and the best approaches to resolving it.

On the other hand, problem resolution in healthcare today cannot be achieved through positional power. People who work in healthcare service delivery tend to develop their culture around service to others. They are influenced little by the legitimate, coercive, and reward types of power that have marked the normal order of business in healthcare organizations. These employees respond to a leader and an organization that foster individual and organizational growth. They appreciate efforts to lead toward service excellence involving quality of care rather than profit maximization. Therefore, positional power is a weak substitute for the personal power of the leader in healthcare service delivery.

### *Influence*

The successful development of personal power allows a leader to use this power to influence people and events. It is through this ability that one is able to accomplish goals. Influencers are needed to move people and organizations into the future before the organization becomes extinct. Innovations are now in demand in healthcare for organizations to survive and thrive, and the creation or revolutionary enhancement of processes, products, services, and so on usually requires some change. As we know, change can be uncomfortable for those who are directly affected by it. In fact, most individuals actively block change even though they may be aware that it is necessary for long-term survival. But the speed of change has become so rapid that many organizations, along with the people who work in them, are at risk for failure.

Those who have developed the ability to influence others understand the value of having clear, compelling, and measurable goals. This recognition is important when attempting to achieve personal goals and becomes all the more vital when leading others to achieve organizational goals. The starting point, then, for becoming a successful influencer is to recognize that the leader must promote in staff the ability to achieve their personal goals. Better yet, if the leader can link the individual's personal goals to the achievement of organizational goals, everyone benefits. Those who have gained the ability to influence others are likely on the path to becoming powerful leaders.

In this time of great disruption in healthcare delivery, the leader must use influence to prepare his staff to exploit change on a continuous basis. The power to influence is an important behavior for almost every employee in a healthcare organization. The industry is being disrupted, and employees of successful healthcare facilities are recognizing the need to change their behaviors (Grenny et al. 2013).

Disruptions usher in a disturbing set of changes for those who have become accustomed to functioning in a certain way that is no longer acceptable. Thus, the healthcare leader must become an expert in the ways to influence these employees to adjust many of their previous behaviors. This effort is difficult to see through to the end because healthcare organizations have numerous separate and distinct occupations, each with its own way of operating that likely has been successful in the past.

The ability to help people change their behaviors can arise from influence (Grenny et al. 2013). Effective leadership requires the capability to foster change through influencing others to move toward a common purpose and goals. Leaders can help staff effect this change through the use of the key leadership skills shown earlier in exhibit 3.1. The use of personal power along with well-developed communication skills can be the recipe for influencing the development of vital behaviors in employees to achieve organizational goals. Also helpful in this effort is to ensure that all employees understand and agree with the purpose of the organization.

## Purpose

The success of an organization can often be attributed to the ability of its leaders to convey exciting and worthwhile future possibilities to its members. The purpose of an organization represents the overarching destination of both individuals and the organization they create, more so than simply generating a profit and supplying jobs for its employees. The purpose becomes the reason the company is in business and the reason employees desire to work there.

Baldoni (2012) argues that leaders must convey a sense of purpose as the central focus of all that is done by the organization and its members. The essential effort behind that purpose is to build a unifying presence.

According to Baldoni (2012), the main purpose of an organization is to bring people together to achieve desired individual and organizational goals. Therefore, leaders must understand how to link individual goals to short- and long-term organizational goals. To be successful as an organizational leader, one must fully appreciate the value of human development in a successful organization. Though this point makes sense to most people, organizations rarely recognize the overwhelming value individuals bring.

The leader can be instrumental in realizing this potential while defining the purpose of the organization. That purpose should certainly be the unifying component of any organization that is delivering services as important as healthcare. However, many healthcare organizations seem to have lost—or never really defined—the meaning of their most important calling. The leaders of those organizations must bring organizational purpose back to their healthcare delivery system.

According to Mourkogiannis (2006), a unifying purpose is crucial for all businesses but is missing from a large number of companies. The first task to be tackled by the leader, with input from the followers who work with the customers, is to develop the organization's purpose and hardwire it into the organizational **culture.** It is one thing to talk about purpose and its importance, but it is another to actually develop a purpose for an organization that has the support of all employees. This is a difficult task, but it must be accomplished.

**Culture**
A way of thinking or behaving in an organization.

Baldoni (2012) argues that an essential purpose of an organization is to shape its vision, which is central to the engagement of employees. The culture of the organization revolves around the mission, values, and vision, and while the culture does not depend on the organization's purpose, it usually is highly influenced by the purpose (Baldoni 2012). Lacking a well-defined purpose that has been accepted by all stakeholders is one major reason some organizations never develop a thick positive culture (discussed later in the book). Whitehurst (2015) takes this connection a step further by linking organizational purpose to employee passion and engagement. In fact, a strong purpose can be instrumental in the creation of a climate of innovation in the organization that will be necessary to achieve its purpose.

Workers in any organization, but especially healthcare delivery, want to feel their work has meaning. If staff believe the work they do is meaningful, they usually become passionate about their share of the work in the organization. Whitehurst (2015) believes that this passion, once ignited, drives employees and, therefore, the organization to exceptional performance. A key leadership skill needed to convey that passion is communication, widely considered to be a prerequisite to reaching consensus on the purpose as a healthcare provider.

## *Goal Achievement*

We end our discussion of the components of leadership with goal achievement because success in the achievement of individual and organizational goals is best gained through the leader's use of the prior components: power, influence, and purpose. In this section, we bring together all the components to address overall goal achievement.

To become an accomplished leader, one must develop a strong understanding of how these components relate to successful leadership in any organization. The components of this advanced leadership development model may help form the answer to the two most important healthcare problems faced today: cost escalation and quality failures. Success in healthcare, or any other industry that relies heavily on employees to deliver services, must pay tremendous attention to both employees and the consumers of the service.

Thus, a vision must be offered as to how to be successful in the delivery of healthcare services to the consumers of these services. This vision or dream must be considered the most important aspect of successful leadership. Its success depends on the development and use of personal power, followed by influence and eventually goal achievement. All members of the organization should buy into the purpose of the organization, as that purpose becomes the guiding force for every step the organization takes on a daily basis to improve the health of its consumers.

For organizational purpose to be that guiding force, the leader needs to spend a great deal of time developing the purpose, as discussed earlier. It is best developed by communicating with the important stakeholders of the organization, including the employees and the consumers, and requires not only talking to them but also listening to what they have to say about their aspirations for the healthcare organization. These individuals know what is being done right and wrong by the facility and can be instrumental in providing advice and guidance for improvement and growth.

The overarching purpose of the modern healthcare delivery system can be distilled into the following achievements: the improvement of health outcomes, a reduction in medical errors, and the delivery of high-quality services by all members of the organization. This purpose can only be achieved if everyone in the organization both understands the purpose and works on a daily basis to fulfill that purpose. The leader must spend much of her time building the service foundation through personal power, influence, and purpose in the achievement of agreed-on organizational goals. This ultimate goal can be achieved through the use of certain leadership skills, as described next.

## Leadership Skills

A bureaucratic organization is designed in a top-down fashion whereby direction flows from the top tip of the organizational pyramid to its wide base. Managerial skills, which typically consist of technical, interpersonal, and decision-making abilities, are usually sufficient to achieve a bureaucratic organization's goals. Here, the manager tasked with accomplishing routine activities is well served if she has learned how to use these managerial skills. Now, however, a wave of disruptive innovation has seized control of the vast majority of businesses in the United States and throughout the world.

Bureaucracies do not perform well in times of rapid change, where decisions have to be made quickly. Bureaucratic organizations are designed to release information from the very top to the lowest levels of the organization on a need-to-know basis. Lower-level employees are not empowered to make decisions without first gaining approval from a manager. This lack of empowerment is not conducive to employee growth and customer satisfaction.

The organizations that are successful in today's accelerated environment have changed to an organic structure with a flattened hierarchy where decisions are made at a lower level than is seen in a bureaucratic structure. With management being replaced by leadership and with empowerment flourishing, a need has emerged for the development of a different leadership skill set. The skills necessary for a decentralized organizational structure are people skills, which for most individuals will take time to learn. Healthcare organizations must make the effort to retrain most, if not all, employees in leadership skills. To become skilled in the use of many leadership skills, one needs to practice them and gain confidence in their application. However, while many organizations offer leadership development programs for all employees, they fail to allow these employees to use the new skills in the course of their work.

The leadership skills necessary for leaders in healthcare organizations include communication skills, empowerment skills, people development skills, and innovation skills. These skills are displayed in exhibit 3.2. They are applicable to any organization but work especially well in service delivery organizations, such as healthcare.

## *Communication Skills*

Communication skills are the main ingredient of charismatic leadership, which, as we have seen, is one of the most important components of personal power. When teaching leadership, convincing students just how important communication skills are in leading others is difficult. Often, managers and leaders believe they have an excellent grasp of communication skills. The problem is that they do not understand that communication requires both talking and listening. Many individuals are good at talking but poor at listening, especially to staff in lower positions, which is problematic when the solution to numerous issues in healthcare delivery requires listening to others to unearth the root cause. In fact, many major challenges found in healthcare delivery today are a direct result of communication difficulties, which have reached epidemic proportions in healthcare.

An essential trait of a charismatic leader is the ability to communicate effectively with employees and customers to convince them of the value of the product or service offered by the business. According to Dubrin (2016), the charismatic leader is capable of communicating the organization's vision in a colorful, imaginative way that is received well and shared by employees in open communication forums. This approach in itself demonstrates the fact that mastery of communication skills is critical for leaders to achieve personal power and become inspirational leaders.

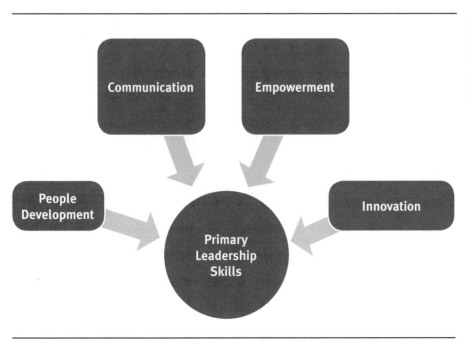

**EXHIBIT 3.2**
Key Leadership Skills for Service Delivery Organizations

Becker and Wortmann (2009) point to the need for a strong culture of communication in the workplace where everyone knows and understands the communication strategy of the organization. In this type of culture, the leader has expended a great deal of time convincing all employees of the value of communicating with each other, with leadership, and with all the customers. The culture of communication also emphasizes the role of listening to others over constantly talking.

As mentioned previously, common practice in a bureaucratic organization is for information to flow from the top of the organization down to lower-level employees. In many instances, this information never reaches all employees in the organization because it may be blocked by managers who believe that withholding information from lower-level employees gives the managers additional power. Another common issue is that messages change many times as they pass from one layer of management to another.

These information flow obstructions cause a disconnect between the leadership of the organization and the employees who deliver services to their customers. It exacerbates already low morale and compromises trust. In most successful healthcare organizations today, communication is rapid, honest, and comprehensive, allowing employees the comfort of knowing that their role is important and valued. Kotter (2014) writes that in times of rapid change, most of the recent research he has reviewed indicates that open communication in an organization is directly related to the success of that organization.

### Empowerment Skills

Empowerment skills involve the ability of leaders to share organizational decision making with employees. They require trust to exist between the leader and the followers, and the only way this trust is gained is if the leader has become a credible force of advocacy for the employees.

Many leaders have difficulty empowering employees, but it must be done to ensure that decisions are made at the lowest level feasible, as rapidly as possible. Often, those in leadership positions talk about empowerment of all employees but fail to enact it. They may be threatened by their followers, which discredits the leader because she fails to model empowerment skills herself. Staff are usually aware that empowerment is only talk and not reality. In these situations, an organizational purpose must be developed that embeds the notion of trust toward power sharing between leader and follower.

Important to note is that when a leader empowers followers, generally the leader is sharing organizational or positional power, not personal power. To share personal power, a leader must engage staff in a leadership development program, allowing them to gain or improve their personal charisma and helping them become expert in particular parts of the work process.

Therefore, true empowerment requires the sharing of positional power, and it is enhanced by providing additional training to staff on an ongoing basis to prepare them to assume future leadership roles.

## People Development Skills

People development skills are critical for the leader who genuinely cares about the growth and development of his staff. Zenger, Folkman, and Edinger (2009) point out that most individuals have within them a strong driving force to improve over time. Effective leaders have the unique ability to foster a positive mind-set in followers that allows them to believe success is possible if they work hard.

If used properly, people development skills can differentiate an average employee from an extremely successful employee. They represent an exciting prospect for both the leader and the followers because these skills set the stage for both to grow in their organizational position. In fact, if applied appropriately, active staff development can inspire followers to the point that they become leaders themselves. Berrett and Spiegelman (2013) note that high-performing leaders can move employees to a much higher level of performance in their achievement of organizational goals than employees might be capable of on their own. This development involves helping employees understand the value of an elevated purpose and providing them with the critical tools to achieve that purpose.

Organizational leaders who are concerned about lower-level employees becoming engaged in the work process should spend time helping them develop the skills and self-confidence necessary for superb job performance. For leaders who develop these skills in followers, no experience is more satisfying than watching employees grow and become increasingly satisfied with their organization and their work. Highly successful leaders are often successful mentors of their staff to help them grow. They care more about the growth and development of their staff than themselves. Berrett and Spiegelman (2013) also argue that superior leaders attract followers who believe that what they do makes a difference in people's lives. This type of leader is sincerely missed when he leaves the organization or retires.

## Innovation Skills

If healthcare services are to be reinvented to reduce costs and improve quality, the effort will require a great deal of creativity and innovation. Dyer, Gregersen, and Christensen (2011) report that in an IBM poll, 1,500 CEOs revealed that creativity was one of the most important competencies for future leaders. The authors discovered that virtually anyone has the ability for innovative and creative thinking. Thiel and Masters (2014) argue that creating new processes, products, services, and so on in a large organization is difficult and is even more difficult for one person. Healthcare organizations, by their nature, are usually too large to have much success with the process of innovation. Thus, it becomes the job of the leader to create a small-scale environment within the business in which innovation and creative thinking can grow, as small size appears to be a major prerequisite for creativity and innovation to occur. The leader with innovation skills also knows to allow a reasonable level of failure to occur; employees are not receptive to taking risks if they expect to be penalized or embarrassed for honest failures.

Bureaucratic organizations do not usually foster creativity and innovation because employees lack trust in their leaders or are limited by a job description that specifies the limits of their responsibilities in the workplace. As organizations grow, they tend to become rigid in their processes and stop seeking change because operations seem to be running smoothly in the current business structure. However, this is the exact time that they should be experimenting with creativity and innovation.

One might think, if only we could take an organization back to when it was first launched and tap all the creativity and innovation involved when it was a start-up. We know this is just a dream, but a number of leadership researchers are pondering how to bring entrepreneurship back to a company that is no longer in the start-up phase and has moved to a bureaucratic structure for control purposes. One of these researchers, John Kotter (2014), believes that a need exists to exploit available opportunities through the creation of a dual operating system housed in the large organization. This new operating system offers the organization opportunities found in the start-up business along with the efficiency and security achieved as a business matures. According to this proposal, the organization is divided into two sections: a traditional hierarchy and a network structure that mimics a start-up in the introductory or entrepreneurial phase of development. This structure offers the organization the best of both worlds in that the hierarchy can concentrate on efficiency and control while the network is empowered to deal with rapid shifts requiring empowered change agents.

According to Dubrin (2016), those who think creatively are capable of both increasing productivity and increasing the size of an existing organization. Innovation requires the actual implementation of the creative thought. Leaders who learned how to think creatively and how to transform their thoughts into innovations have gained one of the most important skills of leadership. Innovation is a key part of the learning organization, an operational framework that supports education, training, and learning continuously throughout the organization. In healthcare, most stakeholders are seeking ways to reduce costs while improving the quality of the services being offered. An in-depth discussion of creativity and innovation is provided in chapter 4.

# Search for the Best Leadership Theory

Many theories about leaders and leadership behavior have been brought forth, with new research emerging every day. Unfortunately, many attempts to explain leadership are essentially refurbished theories with a new spin. This churning of leadership theories is confusing for individuals attempting to learn leadership because of the ever-shifting change in the focus of the newly developed theories written by different authors. Therefore, one rational approach to gaining an understanding of the theory of leadership is to look for themes that remain constant even as new theories come forward, such as the ability to influence others in the collective accomplishment of some predetermined goal.

Leaders usually have a much different approach to goal accomplishment than managers and often rely little on legitimate power in that effort. Their success in goal achievement is a direct result of the support they have gained from their followers, who have agreed on a purpose in what they do at work. It reflects a collective response to organizational and market challenges necessary in today's volatile environment. Effective leaders earn a position from which to lead mainly because they only need to rely on their personal power to attract support from their followers. They use their charismatic qualities to align the purpose of the organization with the intrinsic motivation of their followers (motivation is discussed later in the book). This collective or group response to the leader's vision is critical if that leader wishes to succeed.

Allison (2015) suggests that organizational success is clearly identified through a vision that is communicated to and accepted by all the organization's stakeholders, including the majority of the employees in the organization. If the vision of the leader does not agree with the purpose of the organization, this dissonance can be destructive to the organization and its employees. The leader is responsible for making sure that purpose, culture, and people are in agreement with the way business is conducted. The question then becomes how to determine which theory of leadership and which type of leadership style works best in reforming healthcare organizations while optimizing their most important resource, the individuals who work there.

## *Factors Influencing Choice of Leadership Theory*

According to Lussier and Achua (2016), those who follow leaders who exhibit a charismatic style of leadership are likely to have a great sense of trust and bonding with the leader. This trust and bonding are necessary components for overcoming the tremendous changes facing the healthcare industry into the future, especially when leading highly educated staff, such as physicians, who in many instances are empowering the leader to make decisions for the organization.

One popular leadership style seen in service organizations is transformational leadership. Transformational leaders focus on effecting large-scale change for organizations through their ability to communicate a vision that inspires followers to allow and even seek big changes that secure the vision of the organization (Lussier and Achua 2016).

Among the greatest challenges facing those who are reinventing the healthcare system is shaping the role of physicians. Physicians are obviously key players in the delivery of healthcare, and leaders certainly need physician buy-in as they attempt to solve the dual problems of cost escalation and diminished quality of healthcare services.

Many healthcare systems have successfully used physicians in leadership roles, sometimes at the very top of the hierarchy. According to Schimpff (2012), many senior leadership positions in healthcare systems will be filled by physicians who have received advanced leadership training.

This discussion brings us to one of the most important decisions that must be made by healthcare leaders as the US healthcare system moves through the process of reinvention. What type of training will be offered in the new system to deliver the best return for dollars invested? Obviously, leadership development is a prerequisite for most people working in healthcare delivery today. This training needs to be supplemented with education about how to deal with the process of rapid change and how to turn change into opportunity.

In addition, tremendous pressure is being placed on organizations attempting reinvention to become learning organizations. Bennis and Nanus (2003) argue that the type of learning that is best for an organization depends on the purpose, culture, and ability to absorb the change in the organization receiving the training. They also bring up an important point that needs to be considered by the healthcare organization: Organizations that have become entrenched in their way of doing things need to unlearn or discard completely all knowledge that does not work anymore. This notion applies directly to healthcare delivery systems. For example, healthcare organizations must no longer accept medical errors or hospital-acquired infections as outcomes of doing business. The new rule of business needs to convey that medical errors represent a system failure that needs to be investigated immediately and thoroughly, and efforts need to be put forth to prevent errors from happening. Another example of how to unlearn the behavior has to do with staff being discourteous to patients. Staff must learn that this type of patient treatment will not be accepted. When problems are discovered through communicating with staff and customers on a continuous basis, the solutions must be collectively developed and implemented immediately.

The remaining chapters offer discussion concerning the best leadership style for healthcare organizations as they move from a bureaucratic structure that has always been heavy on management to a more organic structure focusing on leadership and motivation of healthcare employees.

Finally, an interesting point made by Naim (2013) concerns the decay of power that often occurs during times of tremendous change, similar to what we see in healthcare today. He notes that the environment that emerges when change arrives too rapidly for organizations to keep pace is turbulent. He offers several opportunities for individuals who are currently attempting to lead to implement bad ideas. These individuals may use the disruption in the environment to claim simplified solutions to extremely complex problems. They may capitalize on the disruption and fear for their own gain to seize power and make a change that turns out to be disastrous for the organization and its employees. In some cases, by the time they are relieved of their leadership positions, the damage is beyond repair.

## Summary

The way healthcare services are being delivered to a not-so-passive consumer today requires change in both organizational structure and management. To successfully change the structure of the healthcare organization, a movement must take place from short-term management to long-term leadership requiring the empowerment of the healthcare worker. This journey requires leaders, and those who aspire to become leaders, to be identified using an advanced leadership development model.

To build this advanced leadership development model, we focus on the components of leadership that have emerged as among the most common in effective leaders: power, influence, and purpose, ultimately leading to goal achievement. This model must be accompanied by a leader who exhibits personal power and the leadership skills that are necessary for healthcare organizations: communication skills, empowerment skills, people development skills, and innovation skills. This process must be expanded to include leadership development for all members of the organization's workforce.

## Discussion Questions

1. Explain the role of power and influence in the process of leadership.
2. Explain the role of personal power in gaining the support of followers in an organization.

3. What role does the purpose of the organization play in the motivation of the employees of the organization? Explain.

4. Should physicians play a leadership role in the new healthcare delivery system? Explain.

## References

Allison, J. A. 2015. *The Leadership Guide and the Free Market Cure.* New York: McGraw-Hill.

Baldoni, J. 2012. *Lead with a Purpose: Giving Your Organization a Reason to Believe in Itself.* New York: AMACOM.

Becker, E. F., and J. Wortmann. 2009. *Mastering Communication at Work: How to Lead, Manage, and Influence.* New York: McGraw-Hill.

Bennis, W., and B. Nanus. 2003. *Leaders: Strategies for Taking Charge.* New York: Harper Business Essentials.

Berrett, B., and P. Spiegelman. 2013. *Patients Come Second: Leading Change by Changing the Way You Lead.* New York: Greenleaf.

Bolden, R., B. Hawkins, J. Gosling, and S. Taylor. 2011. *Exploring Leadership: Individual, Organizational & Societal Perspectives.* New York: Oxford University Press.

Dobbs, R., J. Manyika, and J. Woetzel. 2015. *No Ordinary Disruption.* New York: Public Affairs.

Dubrin, A. J. 2016. *Leadership: Research Findings, Practice, and Skills,* 8th ed. Boston: Cengage Learning.

Dyer, J., H. Gregersen, and C. M. Christensen. 2011. *The Innovator's DNA: Mastering the Five Skills of Disruptive Innovators.* Boston: Harvard Business Review Press.

Grenny, J., K. Patterson, D. Maxfield, R. McMillan, and A. Switzler. 2013. *Influencer: The New Science of Leading Change.* New York: McGraw-Hill.

Hartford, T. 2016. *The Power of Disorder to Transform Our Lives.* New York: Riverhead.

Kotler, P. 2015. *Confronting Capitalism: Real Solutions for a Troubled Economic System.* New York: AMACOM.

Kotter, J. P. 2014. *Accelerate: Building Strategic Agility for a Faster-Moving World.* Boston: Harvard Business Review Press.

Kuhn, T. 1962. *The Structure of Scientific Revolution.* Chicago: University of Chicago Press.

Lombardi, D. N., and J. R. Schermerhorn Jr. 2007. *Health Care Management.* Hoboken, NJ: Wiley.

Lussier, R. N., and C. F. Achua. 2016. *Leadership: Theory, Application and Skill Development,* 6th ed. Boston: Cengage Learning.

Mourkogiannis, N. 2006. *Purpose: The Starting Point for Great Organizations.* New York: Palgrave Macmillan.

Naim, M. 2013. *The End of Power: From Boardrooms to Battlefields and Churches to States, Why Being in Charge Isn't What It Used to Be*. New York: Basic.

Schimpff, S. C. 2012. *The Future of Health-Care Delivery: Why It Must Change and How It Will Affect You*. Sterling, VA: Potomac.

Thaler, R. H. 2015. *The Making of Behavioral Economics*. New York: W. W. Norton.

Thiel, P., and B. Masters. 2014. *Zero to One: Notes on Startups, or How to Build the Future*. New York: Crown Business.

Whitehurst, J. 2015. *The Open Organization: Igniting Passion and Performance*. Boston: Harvard Business Review Press.

Wilkins, D., and G. Carolin. 2013. *Leadership Pure and Simple: How Transformative Leaders Create Winning Organizations*. New York: McGraw-Hill.

Zenger, J. H., J. R. Folkman, and S. K. Edinger. 2009. *The Inspiring Leader: Unlocking the Secrets of How Extraordinary Leaders Motivate*. New York: McGraw-Hill.

# CREATIVITY AND INNOVATION IN HEALTHCARE

Bernard J. Healey

## Learning Objectives

After completing this chapter, the reader should be able to

- describe the process of developing creativity and innovation in employees,
- discuss the role played by leaders in creating a climate of creativity and innovation,
- explain the differences between intrinsic motivation and extrinsic motivation, and
- summarize the process of innovation.

## Key Terms and Concepts

- Continuous quality improvement
- Creativity
- Dual operating system
- Flow
- Human capital
- Innovation
- Intrinsic motivation
- Network structure
- Reinvention
- Six Sigma

# Introduction

To deal with the dual problems of unsustainable cost increases and poor quality of care, US healthcare organizations are attempting to reinvent the way healthcare is delivered. This is no small task, and many who work in healthcare believe it is impossible to achieve. Reinventing the healthcare delivery system is certainly the greatest challenge to confront the largest industry in the United States since World War II.

The most feasible and effective solution may be the development of **creativity** and **innovation** in every aspect of the healthcare delivery system. This type of change is difficult to effect in a bureaucratic organizational structure run by managers who may block any such shift.

Despite the fact that the healthcare industry is riddled with problems associated with cost escalation and low-quality services, an enormous amount of venture capital remains available to the many businesses and organizations that operate in this field. That availability of money, combined with an industry in the midst of disruption, is encouraging many nontraditional companies to enter a variety of sectors in the healthcare services delivery market. These companies believe they can deliver healthcare services to an increasingly knowledgeable consumer using a new business model. In response, current, traditional healthcare providers should first look at how other markets were disrupted, such as the camera, music, and book markets, to prepare their organization for disruption. At the same time, these incumbents should begin the process of reinventing their particular segment of healthcare delivery.

This type of **reinvention** can only become reality through the emergence of strong leadership supplemented by empowered followers who are not afraid to fail as they innovate. The healthcare leader must spend time and energy encouraging followers to think creatively and pursue innovation, as will be required to reinvent healthcare services in new and redesigned forms, reduce costs, and improve the quality of services.

Stevenson and Kaafarani (2011) argue that for creativity and innovation to bring change for the organization, the leader must understand both concepts as well as the value of each. Creativity is the ability to look at the world, in particular its processes, services, and products, differently than others do. The authors define innovation in terms of three components: "it has to be unique, it has to be valuable, and it has to be worthy of exchange" (Stevenson and Kaafarani 2011, 9).

Furthermore, the innovation, once discovered, must be implemented. Therefore, creative people give us new ways of looking at things, and innovators implement the new ideas.

Individuals tend to be afraid of failure and see no personal value in change; thus, they are not motivated to change. In a way, staff constantly

**Creativity**
The ability to create something new and valuable.

**Innovation**
The creation of new or improved products or services.

**Reinvention**
The activity of making major changes and improvements.

calculate their own cost–benefit analysis of the activities they perform. If in a given movement they are inspired to accomplish a specific goal and the value to them seems greater than the cost, most individuals work in that direction. With that understanding, the leader must create a business environment in which creative thinking can emerge and grow. Before looking at the leader's role in the development of creativity and innovation in the organization, we discuss both concepts in more depth.

# Creativity

As mentioned earlier, virtually anyone has the ability for innovative and creative thinking (Dyer, Gregersen, and Christensen 2011). To elicit that type of thinking in healthcare today, workers must be empowered to use their creativity to find innovative ways to deliver quality services while reducing the enormous waste occuring in the healthcare delivery system. The leader needs to spend time listening to followers and customers to find out what goes wrong and then discover how to fix the problems as a team.

## The Misfit Economy

Clay and Phillips (2015) refer to the presence of a distinct group of misfits in the US economy who are capable of creativity. These individuals have the ability to perform what others may see as miracles in identifying new processes or products and bringing them to fruition. According to Clay and Phillips, these misfits are driven by the opportunity to win their self-designed war with those who have been in the market for a substantial period—an example of intrinsic motivation (discussed later in the chapter)—and are set up to succeed because of an informality mind-set that allows them to avoid the constraints of rules and regulations.

Much insight may be gained from an analysis of how misfits obtain success in existing markets. The misfit mentality frees individuals to think differently. These are the type of entrepreneurs needed to redesign healthcare delivery.

## Concepts in Organizational Creativity

Creativity is all around us, as are creative people who advocate radical, or simply different, ideas or ways of viewing activities, opportunities, obstacles, products, and so on. To think creatively is to use one's imagination to discover deficiencies or gaps in current knowledge. The creative individual is usually defined as someone who can expand her thinking by ignoring rules and regulations in her quest to envision a different future. The end of the creative process typically entails the development of something new and valuable. Creativity in employees has become mandatory for any organization facing the many challenges that healthcare continues to confront in the twenty-first century.

According to Florida and Goodnight (2005), creative employees accomplish the greatest results when they are challenged during the process of work. Creativity can be stimulated by the leader who serves as a role model of creativity for his staff. In addition, all employees must listen to customers and make them part of the creative process.

**Flow**
A mental state in which work is enjoyable, challenging, and ultimately productive.

Csikszentmihaly (2009) points to the development of **flow** in employees' work, which triggers an enjoyable feeling when their work is challenging and the related activities require focus and concentration. Notably, this period of flow also involves a struggle to solve a challenging problem, with individuals expending much energy simply because it is a challenge.

The concept of flow at work is an important revelation for leaders in healthcare organizations because it represents a way to engage employees that is necessary to meet the challenges facing the industry. Csikszentmihaly (2009) points out that the optimal human experience can occur when one's consciousness is characterized as in order. This state can only occur when energy and attention are focused on goals that are realistic and achievable. The leader's responsibility, then, is to help followers achieve their flow, which should ultimately improve healthcare delivery while satisfying the needs of his followers.

**Intrinsic motivation**
Impetus to act found within the individual and driven by internal rewards.

To do so, however, the leader must understand and appreciate the importance of flow and its complementary state, **intrinsic motivation.** Such motivation arises from within, as seen with misfit creatives. Money and status are not always the greatest—and certainly not the only—motivators for healthcare employees. Intrinsic motivation is often the very reason healthcare staff come to work every day. The question becomes how to supply intrinsic motivation to healthcare employees who are undergoing massive change in the way they do their work. The answer is to involve all the employees in the change process from the beginning. The leader needs to tap their expertise in the redesign of the healthcare system where they do their work. The process of change in healthcare is discussed in more detail in chapter 8.

Jim Goodnight, cofounder and CEO of SAS Institute in Cary, North Carolina, has learned how to unleash the creativity of all his company's stakeholders. His research and implementation of certain policies have resulted in unprecedented creativity success, or flow, among SAS employees. He credits his success to the following three principles:

- Keep employees actively engaged by removing distractions.
- Make managers responsible for instilling creativity in employees.
- Engage the customer as a partner in creativity.

Leaders at SAS bring their employees together to facilitate the exchange of ideas and then work to turn the new ideas into innovations. The most important factor is the frequency with which they interact meaningfully with their customers to secure their ideas of how to create better software. SAS refers to this procedure as managing creative capital.

As demonstrated by SAS, stimulating creativity is not necessarily difficult. It does involve empowering employees to view situations, processes, or products in new lights and bringing them together to exchange ideas toward innovation.

Importantly, an idea that is not acted on remains as a thought only. It may even be thought of as a waste of mental energy.

## Creativity in Healthcare: Geisinger Health System

Geisinger Health System, located in central and northeastern Pennsylvania, has been an example of innovative care and payment models for years (Paulus, Davis, and Steele 2008). Geisinger is structured as an open yet integrated delivery system, a type of structure that allows for collaboration. Creativity at Geisinger is fostered through a highly collaborative style of work that incorporates multiple approaches to innovation, including **continuous quality improvement**, **Six Sigma**, and Lean reengineering. Examples of innovations pursued by the Geisinger system are presented in the following paragraphs.

### Personal Health Navigator Program

Geisinger's Personal Health Navigator (PHN) program is a patient-centered medical home designed to provide value for patients through care coordination. Innovators at Geisinger created the concept from an existing process with the goal of ensuring the availability of primary and specialty care 24 hours a day, seven days a week to Geisinger patients. Patients are assigned a dedicated health navigator, who attempts to empower patients to learn more about their health issues and to navigate the healthcare system and then make educated decisions about appropriate health services. This relatively new health initiative was seen as a way to transition a patient from expensive episodic healthcare to a primary care approach. The PHN program, designed to target the elderly Medicare population, was launched in 2006 and has focused on disease management and preventive care (Maeng et al. 2015). This program has achieved savings in total healthcare costs and reduced acute inpatient care. Maeng and colleagues (2015) attribute their success with the program to improved data, enhanced leadership focused on the entire care process, and improved quality of care.

In addition, the program resulted in enhanced patient satisfaction and care accessibility, reduced hospitalization rates, increased use of home-based health monitoring, and improved focus on the proactive management of

**Continuous quality improvement**
An approach to quality in which managers and workers continually strive for improved performance.

**Six Sigma**
A data-driven approach to eliminating defects that sets as a standard no more than six errors per 1 million opportunities (the statistical threshold of 6$\sigma$).

chronic diseases. As the US healthcare delivery system moves to bundled payments and outcomes-based reimbursements, this model is already reducing costs while improving healthcare quality (Maeng et al. 2015).

### Chronic Disease Care Optimization

Geisinger's efforts to optimize chronic disease care for patients with high-prevalence chronic diseases include a program on preventive care. The initiative works toward prevention of the long-term complications that can result from having a chronic disease and not making lifestyle changes.

### ProvenCare Model

Geisinger created a model for treating coronary artery bypass graft (CABG) patients using best practices, developing risk-based pricing, and encouraging patient engagement. Called ProvenCare, this model is based on 40 discrete care process steps for patients undergoing CABG procedures and involves several multidisciplinary teams consisting of Geisinger staff, who developed and implemented the process steps. The workflow includes the delegation of clinical responsibilities to nurses, pharmacists, and medical assistants while ensuring that clerical work is performed by clerks and not clinicians. The steps were hardwired into both human and electronic workflows related to CABG care. In recent years, the ProvenCare program has been expanded to other medical procedures.

As Paulus, Davis, and Steele (2008, 1243) note:

> Geisinger redesign efforts are focused on developing and refining an innovation infrastructure that can adapt to new evidence, efficiently and rapidly translate that evidence into care delivery, and focus on patient benefit in a setting where many or [most] patients would be excluded from randomized trials because of age, comorbidities, and other limiting factors.

## Innovation

Stevenson and Kaafarani (2011) argue that although innovation may be hard to define in the twenty-first century, the US healthcare industry cannot exist as a competitive business without it. McDonald (2013) goes further, saying that innovation is the only real answer to solving the many pervasive problems inherent in the healthcare delivery system. For example, the use of innovative technologies across the entire healthcare sector offers the prospect of a coordinated system of care at a reduced cost to payers.

Innovation involves not only the envisioning of solutions to problems but also the implementation or commercialization of the new idea.

Innovation does not just happen; it usually results from the collective action of team members in the organization.

The starting point for innovation is a creative idea, which can originate anywhere, whether in the organization, often by those who work directly with the current product or service, or from outside the company, coming forth from the user—the customer—of the existing product or service. The innovation process then moves to development of an improved product or service.

## The Innovation Process

Mckeown (2012) points out that to win or sometimes even survive in an age of uncertainty, a business must constantly experiment, learn, fail, and adapt to changing circumstances. He argues that success means adapting to a changing environment and then moving past the constraints of the current situation. Innovations can play a large role in this successful adaptation. Thus, Mckeown (2012) suggests leaders must create a company culture of super-adaptability.

The process of installing an innovation process in a formerly bureaucratic, top-down, management-driven organization is a difficult feat for any leader. But this is exactly the task facing the healthcare leader responsible for improving quality and reducing costs.

The process of innovation usually involves multiple steps, and the effectiveness and value of each step depends on the type of industry in which innovation is being practiced. The most common steps in an innovation process are the following:

- Idea generation
- Idea screening
- Experimentation
- Commercialization

### Idea Generation

The first step, generating ideas, is the most critical because without creativity, few if any new ideas would come from the organization. As mentioned elsewhere in the chapter, the lack of new ideas is a limitation of the bureaucratic structure found in many businesses, especially many healthcare systems.

As indicated by Hill and colleagues (2014), before innovative ideas can flow, leaders need to create an environment in which staff are free to tap their imaginations. Thus, two important roles for the leader in the process of innovation are facilitating employee willingness to do the hard work required for innovation and setting up individuals to succeed at innovation. In short, idea generation requires followers to generate ideas and leaders to create and maintain a location for those ideas to be generated.

### Idea Screening

Innovators also need help from their leader in screening all the ideas that are generated by a motivated team. Screening ideas involves assessing the pros and cons of potential innovations through a selected team of followers led by the manager in a transparent process. By making the screening of ideas a committee-based process, the leader involves multiple people in the process and makes clear to followers that all ideas are valued. Rewards can be attached to ideas that are turned into successful innovations—often, a simple, sincere thank-you and acknowledgment of the success story suffice.

### Experimentation

Numerous experiments must be conducted before the approved innovations move into the commercialization phase of the innovation process. At this point, the leader invites support staff and potential customers to become involved with determining the feasibility of an innovation being adopted by the company. In many instances, a prototype of the new product or service is offered to a small group of employees and potential customers for evaluation. Once all the evaluators and team members are satisfied with the new offering, it can be released for commercialization.

### Commercialization

The commercialization stage is where creative ideas become a work in progress. The leader must make every effort to ensure that the innovation solves a problem or fills a need before the commercialization button is pushed. Once the go-ahead is given in this phase of the innovation process, designated implementers move to make the new product or service available to the market. Commercialization is usually the final stage in the new product process and entails many decisions, including timing of the launch, initial market size, and promotion strategies.

Many businesses have begun to heed the lessons from industries that have shifted due to disruptive innovation, such as the demise of Kodak and Circuit City, to spur creativity among their employees. Examples such as these provide stark and compelling stories to help employees understand how and why their organization might be disrupted and how to deal with disruption as it occurs in healthcare.

### *Bureaucracy and Innovation*

As discussed earlier in the book, bureaucratic organizations with a top-down organizational chart, such as hospitals and health systems, do not usually foster creativity and innovation among their employees. The primary reasons, among many, are a lack of employee trust in managers and bounded job descriptions—stated responsibilities typically do not include "produce new ideas" or "develop new ways of working." As organizations grow, they tend to become rigid in their processes and no longer seek change because the current business structure seems adequate for continued viability. Leaders in static bureaucratic organizations often do not understand the importance of continuous improvement of products or services.

A new business that succeeds soon after beginning operations exhibits all the qualities required for rapid growth, including the following:

- The new owner caters to her customers and employees, recognizing that happy employees tend to remain with the company and satisfied customers tend to return to the company for additional purchases.
- The organizational structure is flat, and the employees are empowered to act on emerging situations, so decisions are made rapidly.
- Customer service is superb.
- Change is viewed as a friend, not an enemy.

As the business grows further, managers are hired and rules and regulations replace common sense. A bureaucracy is created to ensure efficiency and control. The many qualities of a start-up that led to the initial success are lost, and the very growth that perpetuated early success leads to an ultimate decline and, in some cases, bankruptcy.

Most important, the creativity and innovation that gave this company its initial growth and success die. This is the spiral currently seen in the growth of large healthcare systems.

Two possible resolutions capable of reversing this spiral, collaboration and the dual operating system, are discussed next.

## Collaboration

Hill and colleagues (2014) suggest that when problems get complicated or unmanageable, individuals seek collaboration with people from other disciplines to develop innovative solutions. In this effort, the role of the leader is to look inside and outside the organization for advice on the problems. By including the viewpoints of other disciplines, one may see possible solutions to healthcare delivery that would not otherwise be discovered. For example, a surgical unit may view the safety checklist used by aviation crews as a potential solution to medical errors and hospital-acquired infections. Although this tool comes from another industry, its implementation still requires collaboration among different disciplines in the healthcare industry.

## Dual Operating System

According to Kotter (2014), organizations need to exploit available opportunities through the creation of a **dual operating system.** This type of

**Dual operating system**
A structure for running a business under parallel schemes that feature the creativity of a start-up and the efficiencies of a mature business.

operating system provides a means to run parallel business models in the same organization with the creativity, energy, and freedom of a start-up alongside the efficiency and security of a mature business.

Specifically, in a dual operating system, the organization is divided into two sections: a traditional hierarchy and a **network structure** that mimics a start-up in the introductory or entrepreneurial phase of development. This structure offers the organization the best of both worlds in that the hierarchy can concentrate on efficiency and control while the network is empowered to deal with the rapid adjustment required of such change agents (Kotter 2014).

The network structure is entrepreneurial in every sense. It is small in scale, and the limited number of employees operate as a team. Everyone in this network is empowered to use creative methods for finding new ways to perform business activities and discovering new ventures to exploit. Risky ventures that may be avoided in the bureaucratic structure of the organization are tolerated in the network structure, and the concept of failure is non-existent, as each employee is involved in experimentation to allow the venture to succeed. The excitement of a new venture is ever present, building intrinsic motivation in staff.

**Network structure**
A type of operational framework in which employees are empowered to pursue new products or ways of delivering services.

Kotter (2014) argues that this dual organization ushers in the opportunity to exploit the most important duties of managers and leaders. In a dual structure, the managers are expected to do what they do best: guarantee efficiency and stability for the traditional side of the organization. Their role in shoring up efficiencies allows network leaders to concentrate on building a creative team to facilitate required change in a rapidly evolving environment such as that faced by healthcare organizations that are being disrupted by innovation.

### Disruptive Innovation

Dyer, Gregersen, and Christensen (2011) share five skills evident in individuals who are successful at accomplishing disruptive innovation. Among the most important of these is the ability to think differently than others by "connecting the unconnected" in their thought processes. These special innovators support their ability to expand their thinking by gathering information through questioning others. They use this information to network further, expanding their thought horizons. This network both depends on and is enhanced by communication skills, which are a major part of the personal power usually found in successful leaders and empowered followers.

With the healthcare industry now ripe for major changes, creative destruction and disruptive innovation have been unleashed. The concept of creative destruction was outlined by economist Joseph Schumpeter (1936), who posited that old products and services are usually destroyed to create better products and services as replacements.

According to Christensen, Grossman, and Hwang (2009), disruptive innovation has worked well to lower costs and improve quality in many sectors of the business world and is now hard at work doing the same in healthcare. These two forces are producing enormous opportunities—and risk—for anyone working in the current healthcare industry. The word *current* emphasizes the fact that change is under way, and survival usually depends on leaders and empowered followers using creativity and innovation in their collective response to a change in the environment.

Topol (2009), for example, points out that many components of the current healthcare delivery system are on the brink of creative destruction to make room for an improved system that will cost less and enhance the quality of services offered. Hwang and Christensen (2008) argue that disruptive innovation explains why start-up companies, in their attempts to reduce costs and offer more accessible solutions than the incumbent organizations, can consistently out-compete firms that have dominated the market for years. The US healthcare system has been protected by third-party payers and government policy, but that protection is rapidly eroding, making healthcare fair game for disruption by a whole host of start-ups looking for profitable ventures. This erosion in protection has occurred because evaluations completed by government and third-party payers have discovered waste in many parts of the healthcare delivery process.

Many businesses outside of healthcare have accepted disruptive innovation as a challenge that must be met sooner rather than later. The key to disruptive innovation is in challenging knowledgeable employees to think differently, use their creativity to generate new ways of doing things, and make innovation of products and services a daily occurrence. Most organizations have the capability to improve quality consistently while eliminating waste. Once they take these performance improvement measures, they are poised to handle the fluctuations that accompany disruption. Interesting to note is that every part of the healthcare sector, including hospitals, care providers, insurance providers, drug companies, and medical device suppliers, is making attempts to lower costs.

## Development and Motivation of Human Capital

Most bureaucratic organizations worry little about how to motivate their lower-level staff. They tend to place total faith in the traditional model of success whereby all power comes from the top of the organizational structure. As discussed earlier in the book, the sole purpose of this type of structure is to produce efficiency for the organization so that it can make the largest amount of profit possible.

**Human capital**
The collective skills and knowledge of the workforce, including creativity brought by employees to the organization to create value.

In this view, little consideration is given to the **human capital** of the business. The commonly held belief is that employees are lucky to have a job in this turbulent business climate. Bureaucratic healthcare managers tend to forget that lower-level employees are the very individuals who deliver healthcare services to their patients.

Many of these providers are, in fact, highly educated, and most began their careers motivated to offer excellent service to their patients.

However, this motivation may be diminishing for a majority of healthcare staff as the industry has become disrupted and increasingly competitive. Adding to this dissatisfaction for some is that the healthcare technology revolution has replaced some of the human capital and threatens to replace more humans as time goes on.

Considering these developments, an important point, as argued by Hunter (2013), is that future success in healthcare is not found in capital equipment or infrastructure but rather in the creativity and innovative potential of its employees. These attributes can be seen in anyone at any time but usually become evident only when the climate is right. The right climate can be created by the leader when the employees are empowered and believe that they are an important part of the success of the healthcare organization. Therefore, creating healthcare organizations that support creativity is mandatory for survival and future success, and this task is the responsibility of organizational leaders who have the ability to empower a creative workforce.

For leaders to develop the right climate for creativity, they must have a comprehensive understanding of the concept of motivation: What are the primary motivators for healthcare workers? Thaler (2015) suggests the theory of gift exchange, whereby if workers are treated well by their employer, with good wages and good working conditions, the gift will be reciprocated in the form of increased productivity and employee retention. This contingent reward concept aligns with the transactional style of leadership, discussed earlier in the book. It is a workable concept because both the leader and the followers can get what they want through mutual giving.

Pink (2009) argues that individuals are motivated both by extrinsic factors (conditions outside themselves) and intrinsic factors (conditions originating within themselves), and both types of factors must be considered in the workplace. Extrinsic motivation usually comes from salary and benefits. According to Pink, these extrinsic rewards are among the main reasons individuals show up to work, but they only have short-term motivational effects. A pay raise, for example, is only motivational until the worker becomes accustomed to it as her rate of pay.

Intrinsic motivators, on the other hand, come from inside the individual and involve conditions that can improve an individual's self-concept.

Pink (2009) believes that intrinsic factors, such as working on projects that are creative, interesting, and self-directed, may be more motivating for many people than are extrinsic factors. Pink's research strongly supports devoting more attention to intrinsic motivators when dealing with individuals working in service organizations, such as hospitals or health systems, especially concerning professional workers who already receive adequate pay and benefits.

This research also supports the belief by more and more leaders that the best way to engage employees in organizational improvement and redesign is to empower them to help form the change process.

According to Nohria, Groysberg, and Lee (2008), individuals are guided in life by four basic drives or motivators:

- The drive to acquire
- The drive to bond
- The drive to comprehend
- The drive to defend

The drive to acquire consists of our need to acquire scarce goods and explains why we often compare our compensation package with that of others. The drive to bond is demonstrated by feeling proud to be a member of the organization. This drive explains how a culture develops in an organization or a business. The drive to comprehend the world around us shows why challenges in the job are such important motivators for many talented people. Finally, the drive to defend explains why people resist change when they cannot comprehend how it will improve them or their organization.

The fulfillment of these drives in the workplace is vitally important to secure the engagement of employees. If that fulfillment is not met, unsatisfied employees will feel pressure to look for work elsewhere. Nohria, Groysberg, and Lee (2008) suggest that organizations can fulfill these drives through several actions or levers. For example, the drive to acquire can be achieved through a reward system that differentiates good performers from average or poor performers.

Nohria, Groysberg, and Lee (2008) also point out that the key to unlocking motivation is realized when the leader understands his responsibility for satisfying all four drives. This understanding is only acquired when he has more than a superficial knowledge of his employees and learns how best to satisfy these important drives in their workplace. Furthermore, the leader must acknowledge that a motivated workforce has the ability to improve the company's performance. To reach this level of understanding in healthcare facilities requires much communication between the leader and staff on how to improve the organization's performance.

# Creating a Climate for Creativity and Innovation

The climate present in an organization is the ultimate responsibility of the senior-most leader of the organization, the CEO. This environment is a direct reflection of his thought processes and is one of the most important aspects of the creative and innovative potential of the business. Stevenson and Kaafarani (2011) suggest that the CEO, as the individual responsible for establishing the big vision, must secure the agreement of the followers to turn that vision into reality. In doing so, the leader creates the climate of confidence among all the staff in their ability to use their creativity to innovate and grow their company.

A key point about creativity and innovation is that neither activity has been an acknowledged part of employee responsibility in a bureaucratic healthcare system. In fact, it has always been the norm in healthcare to separate the leadership and the top managers from other staff, especially in hospitals. Most healthcare facilities house their administration staff in a separate building or a separate floor from the individuals who deliver healthcare services. This siloing may be a major reason problems in healthcare delivery seem to grow as time goes on. In addition, this separation eliminated most of the opportunity for anyone with authority to be heard by those who deal with daily healthcare delivery issues. Finally, it prevented those employees closest to the patients or consumers from viewing creativity and innovation as important to their jobs. Lower-level employees in bureaucracies have been known to avoid offering suggestions to upper-level managers as a way of staying safe by "leaving their brains at home." Nothing was to be gained by exhibiting creativity, and the threat of danger was invited if one's supervisor was insecure.

## *Tolerance for Failure*

To make the changes that are so necessary to reinvent healthcare delivery systems, administrators and employees must first be willing to take great risks. Furthermore, to ask employees to take a risk, some incentive must be offered. Finally, the manager must be able to convince employees that failure really is acceptable. Such an environment is imperative for staff to believe they can take good risks and not be punished in any way if a failure occurs. To generate this trust-filled climate, the leader needs to appreciate that failures will occur and can serve as a valuable learning process for both the workers and leaders involved in a risky venture. This is not to say that repeated failures should be encouraged; instead, employees must understand that they have the leader's support as they work together to respond to the changing healthcare environment through innovation.

In terms of leadership experimentation through disruptive innovation, Burnison (2011) notes the tremendous courage exhibited by leaders in the face of possible failure, and most seem to be able to draw on some inner strength to push forward on change even though the distinct possibility of failure exists. In fact, Burnison suggests that an absolute lack of fear of failure in employees is a prerequisite for strong leadership. Along with self-confidence, an absence of fear of failure is most likely the catalyst spurring constant change.

But how do leaders instill such a tolerance of failure, whether in themselves or their followers? McChrystal (2015) argues that because change is the new normal, now more than ever we must trust employees to take risks in the projects they develop and implement. Employees in turn must trust their leaders to back them up if they make a mistake in their attempt to please their customer.

Leaders must also forgo micromanagement in a climate that tolerates failure. A manager cannot partially empower staff. Particularly in the delivery of healthcare services, employees rarely have time to clear every movement with a superior. Their empowerment means employees are allowed and trusted to do their job as best they can without interference from above. Managers who are successful at bestowing empowerment have wisely discovered that, because the employees are closest to the customer, they usually know more about the process being implemented than the leader knows.

## Developing Creativity of Employees: The Leader's Role

In addition to the strategies mentioned throughout the chapter, this section discusses specific tactics for developing creativity in employees and the importance of a learning organization to this process. In recognition of the barriers that a bureaucratic organization imposes on creativity, the starting point is to remove rules and regulations, develop a decentralized hierarchy, and support empowerment of and intrinsic motivation in employees. An overarching theme that influences creativity is an environment free of clutter. In this case, clutter is distractions that tend to slow down or eliminate the creative process. Duhigg (2016) reports that several top companies clear 10 to 20 percent of an employee's time each week to work on innovative products or services away from the workplace.

As part of his exemplary leadership in creativity and innovation, Goodnight, CEO of SAS, ensures that the tools employees use at work are up-to-date and that the hassles that can waste the precious time of employees are minimized. If an employee needs updated software to perform his job better, all he needs to do is ask for it. Any obstacles that an employee feels impose a barrier to creativity are typically removed upon request by the employee. The goal is for a creative climate to be the norm at SAS.

Another key component to developing employees' creativity is making room for inspiration. According to Stevenson and Kaafarani (2011), inspiration can open up the entire organization to discovery and provides staff the opportunity to follow an innovation strategy.

Leadership characteristics seen in creative leaders sometimes involve unlearning behaviors. Dubrin (2016) points out that leaders in creativity usually exhibit the following characteristics:

- Knowledge
- Cognitive abilities
- An outgoing personality
- A passion for the task leading to flow in the work process

Bolden and colleagues (2011) highlight one behavior in particular that must be unlearned for leaders to foster creativity: the way they use emotions in their leadership approach. Scientific management theory (discussed earlier in the book) deemed emotionality as irrational and unnecessary in the workplace. In fact, emotionality can be a source of added value because it helps improve the performance of the entire organization. It shows how much employees really care about the success of their organization and becomes contagious to others.

### The Learning Healthcare System

In the not-too-distant past, creative destruction and disruptive innovation were thought to be impossible in the well-protected world of healthcare delivery. Although that protection for the largest industry in the United States is essentially gone, in many ways, the challenge of disruptive innovation is a positive force for improving the long-term health of our population. The changes that need to be made in healthcare delivery, if executed properly, should benefit both consumers and providers of medical care.

Those changes can be brought about when hospitals, health systems, and other healthcare entities shift to a learning organization model. Bennis and Nanus (2003) point out that leaders have the responsibility to help their organization learn how to innovate. To fulfill this imperative, the organization must become future oriented by assessing threats and opportunities and preparing the staff for the changes they see looming ahead. Such a learning organization is flexible and participatory, whereby all employees are able to adapt and be involved. Leaders can help the facility or system prepare for innovative learning by demonstrating the value of taking their creative ideas for change through the process of innovation. They must fully understand that the process of creativity and innovation is a team sport that only improves with the creative genius inherent in an empowered staff.

Mckeown (2012) argues that large organizations, such as those in the healthcare services industry, are ripe for adaptation to a learning organization model. He points out that deliberate adaptation requires three important steps: recognition of the need for adaptation, understanding the adaptation required, and taking the steps required to adapt successfully to the changing environment. In this effort, the leader is responsible for making all followers aware of what successful adaptation looks like in the new world of healthcare services delivery.

An important endeavor for leaders of healthcare organizations is to seek learning opportunities to gain the skills necessary to encourage creativity and innovation among their followers. Reiterating Clay and Phillips's (2015) contention, one can learn a great deal from the misfit economy about the art of creativity and innovation.

## Summary

Creativity and creative people are found in every organization. Creativity is using one's imagination to discover deficiencies or gaps in current knowledge. The creative individual is defined as someone who can expand his thinking beyond the typical connections people make. The current healthcare delivery system is in need of creativity as well as employees who are engaged in the process of innovation.

Innovation involves the envisioning of a new concept that is ultimately implemented. It usually results from the collective action of many individuals in the organization. The starting point for innovation is a creative idea, which can originate anywhere in the organization. The innovation typically includes the development of an improved product or service.

The impending creative destruction of the US healthcare system is expected to result in the building of a better system that will cost less to operate and improve quality. In anticipation of this shift, leaders of healthcare organizations must create an environment in which employees believe they may take risks and not be punished in any way if failure occurs. In turn, employees need to know their creativity is strongly supported by the organization and that innovation, although necessary, can be a risky course to pursue.

Developing the climate for innovation and creativity is the responsibility of the leader. In the healthcare organization, this climate is among the most important aspects of the creative and innovative efforts because it reflects confidence among all staff in the ability to use their creativity to innovate and grow.

Leaders of medical facilities can help their organizations prepare for adopting innovation by creating a learning organization. In this environment, the leader brings her followers to take their creative ideas through the process of innovation.

## Discussion Questions

1. Explain the process of disruptive innovation in the healthcare industry.
2. Explain in detail the value of creative employees in the healthcare organization.
3. What is the major difference between intrinsic motivation and extrinsic motivation?
4. What is the role of leadership in the development of creativity and innovation in a healthcare organization?

## References

Bennis, W., and B. Nanus. 2003. *Leaders: Strategies for Taking Charge.* New York: Harper Collins Essentials.

Bolden, R., B. Hawkins, J. Gosling, and S. Taylor. 2011. *Exploring Leadership: Individual, Organizational & Societal Perspectives.* New York: Oxford University Press.

Burnison, G. 2011. *No Fear of Failure: Real Stories of How Leaders Deal with Risk and Change.* San Francisco: Jossey-Bass.

Christensen, C. M., J. H. Grossman, and J. Hwang. 2009. *The Innovator's Prescription: A Disruptive Solution for Health Care.* New York: McGraw-Hill.

Clay, A., and K. M. Phillips. 2015. *The Misfit Economy: Lessons in Creativity from Pirates, Hackers, Gangsters, and Other Informal Entrepreneurs.* New York: Simon & Schuster.

Csikszentmihaly, M. 2009. *Flow.* New York: Harper Collins.

Dubrin, A. J. 2016. *Leadership: Research Findings, Practice, and Skills,* 8th ed. Boston: Cengage Learning.

Duhigg, C. 2016. *Smarter Faster Better: The Secrets of Being Productive in Life and Business.* New York: Random House.

Dyer, J., H. Gregersen, and C. M. Christensen. 2011. *The Innovator's DNA; Mastering the Five Skills of Disruptive Innovators.* Boston: Harvard Business Review Press.

Florida, R., and J. Goodnight. 2005. "Managing for Creativity." *Harvard Business Review* 83 (7): 124–31.

Hill, L. A., G. Brandeau, E. Truelove, and K. Lineback. 2014. *Collective Genius: The Art and Practice of Leading Innovation.* Boston: Harvard Business Review Press.

Hunter, G. S. 2013. *How Innovative Leaders Drive Exceptional Outcomes.* San Francisco: Jossey-Bass.

Hwang, J., and C. Christensen. 2008. "Disruptive Innovation in Health Care Delivery: A Framework for Business Model Innovation." *Health Affairs* 27 (5): 1329–35.

Kotter, J. P. 2014. *Accelerate: Building Strategic Agility for a Faster-Moving World.* Boston: Harvard Business Review Press.

Maeng, D., N. Khan, J. Tomcavage, T. Graf, T. D. Davis, and G. D. Steele. 2015. "Reduced Acute Inpatient Care Was Largest Savings Component of Geisinger Health System's Patient-Centered Medical Home." *Health Affairs* 34 (4): 636–44.

McChrystal, S. 2015. *A Team of Teams: New Rules of Engagement for a Complex World.* New York: Penguin.

McDonald, K. C. 2013. *Innovation: How Innovators Think, Act and Change Our World.* Philadelphia, PA: Kogan Page.

Mckeown, M. 2012. *Adaptability: The Art of Winning in an Age of Uncertainty.* Philadelphia, PA: Kogan Page.

Nohria, N., B. Groysberg, and L.-E. Lee. 2008. "Employee Motivation: A Powerful New Model." *Harvard Business Review* 86 (7): 78–84.

Paulus, R. A., K. Davis, and G. D. Steele. 2008. "Continuous Innovation in Health Care: Implications of the Geisinger Experience." *Health Affairs* 27 (5): 1235–45.

Pink, D. H. 2009. *Drive: The Surprising Truth About What Motivates Us.* New York: Riverhead.

Schumpeter, J. A. 1936. *The Theory of Economic Development*, 2nd ed. Cambridge, MA: Harvard University Press.

Stevenson, J., and B. Kaafarani. 2011. *Breaking Away: How Great Leaders Create Innovation That Drives Sustainable Growth and Why Others Fail.* New York: McGraw-Hill.

Thaler, R. H. 2015. *The Making of Economics: Misbehaving.* New York: W. W. Norton.

Topol, E. 2009. *The Creative Destruction of Medicine.* New York: Basic.

# HEALTHCARE ENTREPRENEURSHIP

Jeff Helton and Nancy Sayre

## Learning Objectives

After completing this chapter, the reader should be able to

- discuss the significance of entrepreneurship in the delivery of healthcare services,
- define the concept of innovation in the context of healthcare delivery,
- describe the types of entrepreneurs that have emerged in healthcare services, and
- understand where entrepreneurship can occur in the current healthcare environment.

## Key Terms and Concepts

- Biomedical entrepreneurship
- Design thinking
- Entrepreneurial innovation
- Entrepreneurial success
- Entrepreneurship

- Innovation approach
- Phase-gate process
- Price sensitivity
- Technological enabler
- Value proposition

## Introduction

The traditional approaches to delivering healthcare services are no longer affordable or sustainable. Different ways of thinking, targeted technology, new methods of management, and unconventional solutions all could lead to profoundly needed innovation.

Although entrepreneurial changes in healthcare have not always led to improvements that lowered prices paid by consumers, improved efficiency in delivering healthcare, produced outstanding quality of care, or made services available to more consumers, opportunity abounds and entrepreneurs are needed in these turbulent times. To the extent that entrepreneurs can disrupt the current state of healthcare, not only can the system improve but also the financial and intrinsic rewards for improving care can be significant.

How can innovation help healthcare deliver services with more value for patients in a cost-effective and efficient method? In this chapter, we discuss entrepreneurship and its role in healthcare innovation.

## What Is Entrepreneurship?

**Entrepreneurship**
A way of creating wealth with a new business innovation.

**Entrepreneurship** as a concept emerged in the 1700s to describe risk-taking or risk-bearing activities. Originally developed by economists, this view presented entrepreneurship as a means of creating new wealth (Drucker 1993). In a more general sense, entrepreneurial activity involved innovation to create some new factor or exploit some perceived opportunity in the economy. An early economics text—Schumpeter's (1936) *The Theory of Economic Development*—explained the process of entrepreneurship as an activity aimed to exploit one of five types of economic opportunity:

- Introduction of a new product, development of a new service, or change in the quality of an existing product or service
- Introduction of a new method of producing an existing good or service
- Opening of a new market to an existing product or service sold elsewhere in the economy
- Development of a new source of supplies or production inputs used to bring an existing product or service to market
- Creation of a new organization to market or produce either an existing or a new product or service

However, the economist's description of entrepreneurship leaves out much of the essence of creating a new economic entity from scratch, as well as the challenges presented to the entrepreneur by environmental factors in the overall economy. Timmons (1989) defines entrepreneurship as "the ability to create and build something from practically nothing." This definition captures the ability of an entrepreneur to identify a business opportunity where others do not, design and build an organization to meet that business opportunity, assess the extent of personal and organizational financial risk, and ultimately create an organization that best mitigates those risks and brings a new business venture or entity to market (Timmons 1989).

As a part of this definition, entrepreneurship must consider how exist-ing resources can meet a business opportunity to identify gaps in existing organizational capacities that preclude a new business venture from going to market. Some factors to be considered include the external regulatory and financing environment, existing capacity in the economy, existing technology or competitor abilities, skills and talents of individuals in that sector of the economy, and factors of production already a part of that market. The suc-cessful entrepreneur is one who can find the optimal solution among these disparate and sometimes conflicting factors (Kuratko and Hodgetts 1998). Exhibit 5.1 illustrates how these factors come together to create an opportu-nity for **entrepreneurial innovation.**

Today's healthcare industry could certainly be considered to have all these factors in play. As elaborated in the next section, changing reimburse-ment rates, questions of efficiency in delivering care, challenges in obtain-ing properly trained labor resources, inefficient distribution of healthcare resources, and numerous other variables all contribute to opportunities for entrepreneurship.

**Entrepreneurial innovation**
Consists of new ways to innovate resulting in greater wealth creation.

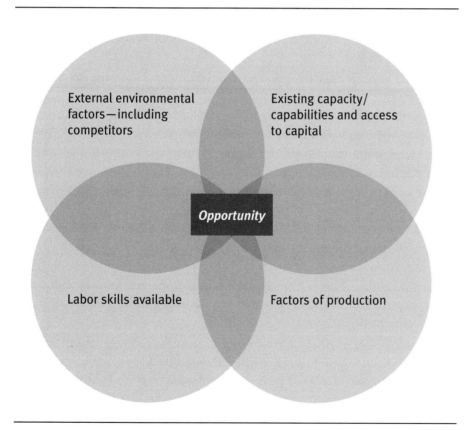

**EXHIBIT 5.1**
Factors Creating an Entrepreneurial Opportunity

External environmental factors—including competitors

Existing capacity/ capabilities and access to capital

*Opportunity*

Labor skills available

Factors of production

## Opportunities for Entrepreneurs in Today's Healthcare System

Drucker (1993) and Asoh and colleagues (2005) identified seven windows of entrepreneurial activity and opportunities for transformation in the healthcare industry:

- *Growth in new knowledge*—Innovations that advance the knowledge of diagnosis and treatment of illness and injury will remain a high priority to improve success in treating healthcare conditions that are currently beyond the capabilities of medical technology.
- *Consumer desires*—The healthcare industry continues to see growth in consumerism as information about healthcare services and treatment options becomes increasingly available. As consumers become better informed, their expectations for efficiency, low cost, and high quality increase.
- *Changes in the industry structure*—As financing and reimbursement mechanisms change, innovation will be necessary not only in technology and products but also in the actual organization and the delivery of healthcare to preserve financial viability for many hospitals and health systems.
- *Aging of the population*—As the population gets older, the need for healthcare services will certainly increase. In addition, as technology lengthens life expectancy, consumers will demand technologies that allow them to lead a more active older life.
- *Process improvement*—As healthcare has become more competitive, a traditional economic model suggests that a business must innovate in ways to improve efficiency and thus reduce price to gain market share. Innovations that promote operational efficiency have been slow to be adopted in healthcare for a variety of reasons, including the presence of persons in the healthcare system with a vested interest in maintaining the status quo (keeping existing relationships for personal or professional gain), a lack of incentives to change processes, and regulatory barriers to deviating from traditional treatment models.
- *Shortcomings in service delivery*—Past initiatives to promote efficiency in healthcare delivery have led to a standardized approach to delivering healthcare services. However, this standardization has led to an increase in consumer dissatisfaction. Calls for more customized, consumer-specific solutions to individual healthcare needs continue, expanding the already significant opportunity for entrepreneurship in the industry.

- *The uncertain nature of the healthcare system*—The healthcare system today is undergoing a great deal of change as patients and regulators struggle with the fact that healthcare is consuming an ever larger part of the US economy. With such growth, access to healthcare is not affordable to many, which brings about myriad changes, such as reductions in payments to healthcare providers and shifts in the manner in which services are delivered—such as a move from inpatient to outpatient care settings for some surgical procedures. Political changes tend to vary toward and then away from healthcare as a priority, which can make access to government funding for innovation or payments from government insurance programs unpredictable. Because private insurers tend to follow the decisions of government insurers, this uncertainty of payment for new services can be compounded.

Ackerly and colleagues (2009) note three broad sectors in the healthcare economy where entrepreneurial ventures may be attractive to investors or to existing businesses seeking a market advantage: pharmaceutical and biotechnology products, medical devices, and healthcare services (such as a new type of care delivery like a freestanding emergency room). In particular, PricewaterhouseCoopers (2000) identified the medical device sector as attractive to entrepreneurs given the availability of capital and increased investment in healthcare services, such as long-term care, home health and telemedicine, and services for the aged. These areas continue to address current needs for service improvement in the industry and as such represent opportunities for today's healthcare entrepreneur.

### Who Are the Entrepreneurs in Healthcare?

Of course, not everyone who attempts to be an innovator in healthcare is successful as an entrepreneur. This section describes some common characteristics of entrepreneurs in the healthcare industry.

The following behavioral traits are seen as particularly relevant to successful entrepreneurship:

- Tendency to seek opportunities for personal achievement
- Inherent management or leadership skills
- Ability to facilitate idea generation alone or in groups
- Ability to sell
- Ability to demonstrate, or designate responsibility to someone who has demonstrated, sound financial management practices

These characteristics are strong predictors of one's ability to found a new business or identify a business venture, develop a reasonable business plan, and identify and implement a new business innovation, with the strongest being high personal achievement and inherent leadership skill (Asoh et al. 2005). These two traits are essential to the ability to form and build teams, facilitate idea generation, and develop salesmanship to not only promote a product but understand the financial business case to create a compelling story for selling the idea to investors (to generate investment resources) who can fund the new venture.

Interestingly, nurses seem particularly disposed to achieving success in healthcare entrepreneurial activities. Nurses tend to readily identify opportunities to improve healthcare services through a process change or see a need for a new product to help them take care of their patients (Asoh et al. 2005). Through their training, nurses become skilled in finding ways to address patient care needs by looking at the bigger picture of a patient's clinical condition rather than a specific characteristic or situation. In addition, nurses tend to have a high commitment to serving patients, demonstrated by the ability to stay in touch with the needs of their customer. They also typically exhibit a level of comfort with risk taking, again in the context of seeking out what is needed to take care of patients. Many nurses also tend to be assertive and skilled in leading patient care teams and can readily translate those traits to **entrepreneurial success** (Roggenkamp and White 1998).

**Entrepreneurial success**
The extent to which an individual is effective in the process of wealth creation.

Certainly, nurses are not the only successful entrepreneurs in healthcare. However, the traits of assertiveness, creativity, leadership, and commitment to patient care tend to be common among nurses and thus are predictors of successful entrepreneurship in the healthcare industry. When looking for successful entrepreneurs—or assessing one's own entrepreneurship potential—attention to the presence or absence of these types of characteristics can indicate an individual's potential success as a healthcare entrepreneur.

Physicians also have started many successful companies in the healthcare sector. DocbookMD is just one example of physicians launching a company out of a recognized need for secure mobile communications with patients. Physicians have also been successful in establishing large corporations, such as Prime Healthcare Corporation, which, as of this writing, owns or operates 42 hospitals in 14 states. Physicians in many market areas have successfully opened hospitals or ambulatory surgery centers, which by federal law must operate with restrictions to prevent physicians from steering patients to facilities that provide them with additional income for a referral. Other physician-owned entrepreneurial companies include medical device distributors, medical malpractice insurance companies, medical software application companies, and physical therapy clinics.

### Where Can Entrepreneurship Occur in Healthcare?

Some readers may think of entrepreneurship as creating business ventures or new companies, and they are correct to an extent. However, entrepreneurship also exists in organizations. In fact, organizations that foster entrepreneurship from within may be among the most successful, as seen later in this chapter with Kaiser Permanente. Internal entrepreneurial ventures in that organization have developed innovations such as new tools in medication administration tracking and improvements in hospital care coordination with other levels of the healthcare continuum.

The increasingly competitive healthcare marketplace creates great opportunity for existing organizations to adapt, meet, and exploit competitive situations for changes in the environmental landscape. A successful entrepreneur may lead teams that develop new community services, such as a healthcare clinic for the homeless population to prevent hospital readmissions or a new information system that tracks patient wait times in the emergency department to improve customer service. The closer interaction now being seen between hospitals and post-acute care providers may also represent an opportunity for an entrepreneurial venture in an organization, perhaps to develop new technologies to facilitate coordinated care among different levels of healthcare, reducing costs and potentially increasing reimbursement for all parties.

An entrepreneur can be just as successful working in an existing organization to lead its change or improvement process as she can starting up a new business venture. Entrepreneurship in healthcare can happen in any manner it could in any other industry—when an opportunity exists in a market or an organization to change a product or create a new service offering. This is an important consideration for current and future leaders in healthcare. Knowing how, when, where, and potentially who can lead an entrepreneurial innovation can be as big a contributor to success as actions to negotiate new payment rates or reduce operating costs.

# Innovation and Entrepreneurship

Innovation starts when someone creates an idea that brings value or perceived benefit either to the stakeholder(s) or customers. The process of implementing the product or service begins after the idea has been investigated and considered viable. Assuming implementation is successful, the final step is to take the innovation to the market.

Innovation consists of the search, discovery, experimentation, and development of a new product or service, and entrepreneurs are the people who organize and manage a new enterprise, usually with considerable initiative and risk. Innovation can be incremental—representing a modification to existing technology or products—or disruptive, such that it introduces an entirely new way of doing things in a product or market (Garrety, McLoughlin, and Zelle 2014). First, we provide a brief overview and history of innovation and describe the innovation process; in a later section, we discuss disruptive innovation in more depth.

**Biomedical entrepreneurship**
Activity that produces new medical devices, drugs, and medical treatments.

According to Arlen Meyers (2015), a physician entrepreneur, health entrepreneurship is about creating value in digital health products or services or developing new healthcare delivery or business processes, services, or platforms. **Biomedical entrepreneurship**, for example, refers to commercializing drugs, devices, biologics, vaccines, diagnostics, or related products.

Innovation in technologies, applications of medical knowledge, and types of patient services has been occurring in medicine for centuries. For example, antisepsis, anesthesia, and the emergence of public hospitals were significant advances in the late nineteenth and early twentieth centuries. The advent of public health insurance in the form of Medicaid and Medicare and the concept of medical records in the 1960s as well as the introduction of CT (computed tomography) scanning in medical practice in the 1970s are just a few examples of innovations that have significantly contributed to progress in medicine. They all required a visionary with a great idea to start those technologies and modifications on their way to adoption in medical care.

Innovation in healthcare has never been easy. Considerable forces, such as public policy, funding for development, competition from existing technology, accountability for patient care outcomes, multiple stakeholders, and a convoluted purchasing process, are current influences that push against innovation (Herzlinger 2006). The many industry players in healthcare have considerable power and influence. The American Medical Association is among the top five largest lobbying groups in the United States (Center for Responsive Politics 2016). It exists to advocate for the interests of physicians and regularly opposes innovations that may threaten the role of or payment to physicians. Similarly, hospitals, insurers, personal injury attorneys, and population and patient segments (e.g., AARP for seniors) have their own agendas that either promote or oppose innovations in healthcare. The complex system of payments, mostly from third-party payers (i.e., not the patient); the extended investment of time and resources for developing new products or services; the enforcement of federal and state rules and regulations; and the influence of physicians in health decision making can impose complications on the process of innovation. As Herzlinger (2006) notes, "The friends or foes lurking in the healthcare system . . . can destroy or bolster an innovation's chance of success."

Despite—or perhaps as a result of—the obstacles, the US healthcare system is ailing and in need of innovation and entrepreneurship. Information technology, new healthcare delivery settings, new financing mechanisms, and new treatment procedures and equipment all represent areas where innovation and an entrepreneurial approach can yield benefits to the contemporary healthcare economy.

### Making Innovation Happen

Going for a walk, writing dreams down, embracing serendipity, listening to those in other organizations, borrowing from other industries, recycling ideas from the past, cultivating hunches, pursuing gut feelings, or reading the ideas of great authors are some of the ways individuals come up with that "Eureka!" moment that launches a great idea. Of course, customers often offer meaningful and viable suggestions for product enhancements or spin-off products, but so can the supply vendor, the landlord, the accountant, or the delivery person. In addition, employees are often overlooked as a source of innovation, despite the fact that they are among the greatest fonts of wisdom about a company's products or services. A suggestion box and the occasional brainstorming session have been known to release new ideas from employees; however, newer approaches, such as design thinking, innovation teams, methodical idea generation, product screenings, and new product launches are being implemented by forward-thinking organizations to yield promising innovations on a regular basis.

**Design thinking** is a methodology by which to develop new human-centered products, services, spaces, and systems. It is a structured way to devise solutions with the intent of an improved future result. It also is a form of creative, solution-focused thinking—starting with a goal instead of solving a specific problem. The process involves the following stages:

> **Design thinking**
> A method for designing new human-centered products and services.

- Inspiration
- Goal or problem clarification
- Interviewing or data collection
- Concept generation
- Result synthesis
- Iterative prototyping with feedback

Successful solutions, such as a low-cost device for treating jaundice in infants in developing nations or a scalable system for providing affordable eye care, have relied on this approach, which has been championed by IDEO (www.ideo.com/work/openideo). Kaiser Permanente, a large integrated health system serving the health needs of 8.6 million individuals across the United States, has implemented an internal design-thinking innovation methodology and a consultancy team to cultivate, refine, and implement innovation in the organization. This **innovation approach** is aimed at developing increasingly efficient ways to perform high-value activities, usually associated with patient care. For example, Kaiser Permanente has developed a process to reduce medication errors and a method for nurses to exchange patient knowledge quickly and reliably, gaining a distinctive internal innovation methodology in the process. Change is fully embraced (McCreary 2010):

**Innovation approach**
A method of designing new, increasingly efficient ways of delivering healthcare to patients.

> Every Innovation Consultancy project [at Kaiser Permanente] includes a "change package"—a set of detailed, clearly written guidebooks that fully describe the innovation, the reasoning behind its creation, the process by which it was developed (with shout-outs to staffers who participated), the benefits it's meant to produce for patients and staff alike, user testimonials gathered during pilot implementations, and the metrics that will be used to evaluate its performance over time.

Regardless of the way an idea emerges or how healthcare innovation is defined or characterized, entrepreneurs can come from within an organization, such as Kaiser Permanente, or be found outside the industry altogether, such as the founder of Oscar, a new health insurance company self-described as "Simple health insurance, smart healthcare," who came to the healthcare industry from the investment finance world (Lamantia 2015). The lone inventor in his garage, epitomized by Bill Gates of Microsoft or Bill Redington Hewlett and Dave Packard of HP, is a popular symbol of US entrepreneurism. More typically, entrepreneurs are organization-based individuals relying on their social context, within which they acquire many psychological and social resources necessary to create new organizations (Audia and Rider 2005). No matter who delivers the idea, once it emerges and seems worthwhile to pursue, a systematic process of evaluation should occur to convince the entrepreneur, organization, or funder of the potential for success. An example of such a systematic process is the phase-gate process described later in this chapter.

## Current Challenges to Entrepreneurship and Innovation in Healthcare

Hwang and Christensen (2008) present several factors that impose limits on entrepreneurial innovation in healthcare. The fragmented nature of the healthcare system, in which multiple types of providers deliver different elements of healthcare, makes implementing a reasonable solution—one that addresses the many needs in the US healthcare system—difficult. An improvement in one part of the healthcare system may take away benefit from another part of the system and thus create a barrier to full adoption of an innovation. For innovation to take hold and improve on the inefficient, poor-quality outcomes often achieved by the US healthcare system, some benefit must be gained by all participants. Otherwise, resistance will be encountered that may stall a promising innovation. Another variable is the fact that the type of innovation that could disrupt the norm in healthcare and provide a substantial improvement requires a market in which consumers are willing to put their money where they see the greatest value (Guo 2003; Martin 2011). The financing of healthcare services using health insurance and its third-party payer system takes away the typical economic incentives we might see in other sectors of the economy, such as consumer products. Also, the fact that the healthcare system is so fragmented does not diminish the interdependencies of these elements; changing only one part of the healthcare system without addressing these interdependencies may cause an innovation to fail.

The prevalence of healthcare regulations also potentially limits entrepreneurship in the industry. While some observers may argue that the presence of these regulations protects the vested interests of participants already in the marketplace, entrepreneurs in the healthcare field will be on the defensive to prove the safety and efficacy of their innovation in that market. In fact, regulations create a degree of inertia that slows entrepreneurial innovation and may preserve inefficient and high-cost service delivery. Similarly, the linkage of payment for healthcare services to regulatory approval cannot be discounted. Under the current system, new technologies must gain regulatory approval prior to being reimbursed by insurers. Thus, the entrepreneur has a significant stumbling block. An innovation may be ready for market but not able to be sold because of the need to prove its safety and efficacy before regulatory approvals can be obtained. The current approach by government insurance programs and commercial insurance plans, whereby payment rates per unit of service are continually reduced, should represent an incentive for innovation and an attractive opportunity for entrepreneurial ventures. However, the downward push on per unit payments may limit the amount of capital available in that segment of the market and make funding such innovations unattractive to outside investors.

## Taking an Idea to Implementation

A **phase-gate process** is a project management technique that divides the process from idea to implementation into phases with decision points called gates. At each gate, the decision to continue in the process is made by a manager, committee, task force, or management team on the basis of information available at the time, including the details required for each phase of the process. Typically, the phases include ideation, scoping, building a business

**Phase-gate process**
A way to divide a process into steps that move from idea to implementation.

**EXHIBIT 5.2**
Idea Generation
and Screening
Process

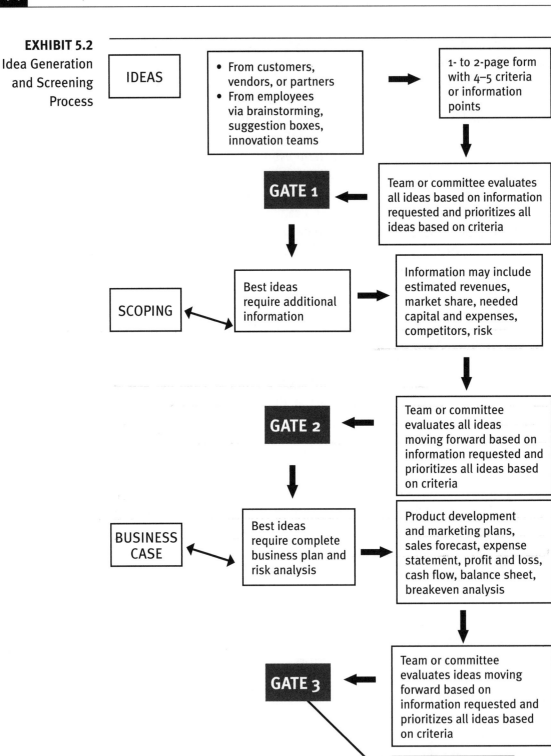

IDEAS

- From customers, vendors, or partners
- From employees via brainstorming, suggestion boxes, innovation teams

1- to 2-page form with 4–5 criteria or information points

**GATE 1**

Team or committee evaluates all ideas based on information requested and prioritizes all ideas based on criteria

SCOPING

Best ideas require additional information

Information may include estimated revenues, market share, needed capital and expenses, competitors, risk

**GATE 2**

Team or committee evaluates all ideas moving forward based on information requested and prioritizes all ideas based on criteria

BUSINESS CASE

Best ideas require complete business plan and risk analysis

Product development and marketing plans, sales forecast, expense statement, profit and loss, cash flow, balance sheet, breakeven analysis

**GATE 3**

Team or committee evaluates ideas moving forward based on information requested and prioritizes all ideas based on criteria

Product development, testing, and launch

case with risk analysis, development, testing and validation, and launch. This process provides a road map for moving a project along to decrease the time to implementation and improve the likelihood of success. A typical phase-gate process is outlined in exhibit 5.2.

In healthcare, new ideas can come from patients or their families, clinicians, hospital employees, vendor partners, or the public. At Yale-New Haven Hospital (YNHH), an online program called WorkSMART allows staff members to submit ideas online (www.weareynhh.org/worksmart.html). A committee reviews the ideas, and feedback from the committee is communicated directly to the employees whose suggestions have been accepted. Most important, those employees are recognized and rewarded. The goal of WorkSMART is to cut waste and improve cost-effectiveness. In its first year, almost 700 employees contributed 1,200 ideas that saved YNHH more than $700,000.

This example demonstrates that a suggestion box is no longer adequate to capture employees' ideas. <u>Organizations and managers should enthusiastically and methodically solicit new ideas through established programs if they expect to innovate</u>. Many organizations have created a short form (one to two pages) to collect ideas and relevant information. A committee, task force, or management team sets the criteria for passing through this gate to the scoping phase. Adherence to criteria may be assessed by asking questions such as the following:

- Is the idea consistent with the mission, vision, and goals of the organization?
- Is the idea aimed at the existing or a new client base?
- Does the idea confer revenue generation or cost savings?
- Is the idea unique?

The evaluating team ranks and prioritizes the idea using a scoring rubric. Some organizations weigh the importance of each criterion. Whether an absolute number must be achieved to pass to the next stage or only the top two or three ideas are selected to proceed must be established in advance of screening ideas.

Some parameters that may be examined in this phase are estimated operating expenses and capital, estimated revenues or market share, reimbursement issues, US Food and Drug Administration or other regulatory approvals, competitive forces, required skill sets, and issues of intellectual property or other legal challenges. Evaluation of some of these parameters may be postponed to the business case phase, but the information needed and the scoring parameters are set in advance of passing the scoping gate. Exhibit 5.3 provides an example of a scoring rubric to pass gate 1 illustrated in exhibit 5.1.

EXHIBIT 5.3
Scoring Rubric
for Gate 1

| Criteria | Idea 1 | Idea 2 | Idea 3 | Idea 4 |
|---|---|---|---|---|
| | *Score × Weight = Weighted score* | | | |
| **Criterion 1:** Consistent with mission, vision, and goals of the organization Score 1–10 Weight: 0.40 | 3 × 0.40 = 1.2 | 6 × 0.40 = 2.4 | 8 × 0.40 = 3.2 | 4 × 0.40 = 1.6 |
| **Criterion 2:** Aimed at the existing or new client base Score 1–10 Weight: 0.25 | 6 × 0.25 = 1.5 | 8 × 0.25 = 2.0 | 8 × 0.25 = 2.0 | 6 × 0.25 = 1.5 |
| **Criterion 3:** Confers revenue generation or cost savings Score 1–10 Weight: 0.25 | 4 × 0.25 = 1.0 | 8 × 0.25 = 2.0 | 8 × 0.25 = 2.0 | 4 × 0.25 = 1.0 |
| **Criterion 4:** Uniqueness Score: 1–10 Weight: 0.10 | 8 × 0.10 = 0.8 | 5 × 0.10 = 0.5 | 8 × 0.10 = 0.8 | 5 × 0.10 = 0.5 |
| **TOTALS** | **4.5** | **6.9** | **8.4** | **4.6** |

In this example, four ideas are compared using the scoring rubric, and the analysis of these ideas across four evaluation criteria helps identify which ideas should move further into the development process. The four criteria are consistency with the organization's mission, expansion of client base, increased revenue or reduced expense (aimed at improving profitability), and uniqueness (aimed at differentiating ways to garner market share or maintain profitability). Uniqueness may be a valuable characteristic in representing an innovation that expands on or diverts from prior ways of accomplishing organizational goals and could ultimately result in a new market niche.

Those ideas that are ranked highly go on to the scoping phase, where more detailed information is required. So, using the example of scoring in exhibit 5.3, idea 2 and idea 3 might be further evaluated. That additional evaluation might include detailed estimates on revenues or expense savings, opportunities to grow or expand the business, presence or proximity of competitors offering similar products, the relative strengths and weaknesses of the firm to offer or produce the new idea, or the possibility of regulatory or legal hurdles to overcome. Such an evaluation must be detailed to substantiate any rationale proposed about the future viability of a business venture.

Once these data have been gathered for this next level of evaluation, a team or committee may evaluate them using a rubric similar to that shown in exhibit 5.3. At any point that the facts appear to not support a new venture, the organization may decide to discontinue pursuing that idea without further consideration.

Ultimately, one or two good ideas may survive to the next step in the process, development of a detailed business case or business plan. Such a business plan includes the following:

- A detailed description of the product or service envisioned by this new venture
- Comparison of the proposed venture with other similar competitors, describing the relative strengths and weaknesses of this venture vis-à-vis the competition
- Detailed plans on implementation for production of the new venture's product or service, including the estimated capital requirements, production resources required, and expected output volumes from the venture
- Identification of managers or executives to lead the venture, including definition of management roles and responsibilities and description of their qualifications to carry out such roles and responsibilities
- A detailed financial plan identifying expected revenues, operating expenses, and profits, as well as an estimate of cash flows needed to fund or repay any capital investment in this venture

Once the idea has progressed this far in the phase-gate process, managers and potential investors must conduct a thorough risk analysis of the proposed venture. For the analysis to be performed, the business plan must be evaluated to identify essential business functions or processes that, *consequence* if interrupted, would cause the business venture to be unable to operate as planned. This assessment should also include a description of any resources the business venture could not do without or regulations that, if changed, may prohibit continued operation of the venture. Examples of such factors are natural disasters, accidents, utility failures, discontinuation of operation by suppliers, an economic downturn that affects demand for services, changes in the labor market that create workforce shortages, and changes in healthcare licensing regulations.

Knowing the factors that can influence the success of a business venture can help managers carry out the next step in this evaluation process—a risk assessment. The risk assessment should determine the likelihood of adverse events happening and attempt to place a value or cost on those events should they occur. For example, if the success of a new business venture relies on a specific type of supply, are alternative vendors in the market that can meet that supply needed, and if so, what impact would the switch have on operating expenses, inventory requirements, and cash flow?

Some observers liken this type of assessment to an expected value analysis, and the parallels are significant. Essentially, this risk assessment creates a probability-weighted value for a potential adverse outcome. Some risks are of such low probability of occurrence or would have such a minimal impact on the venture as to require only a notation to acknowledge their existence. Other risks may be frequent enough or severe enough to result in an adverse financial impact that the risk must be mitigated before a project can continue. A potential innovation must be fully assessed for risk; that risk must be quantified; and, to the extent possible, steps must be taken to reduce either the probability of an adverse event or the extent of loss from such an event. This may be the point at which a project cannot proceed and the evaluation process starts anew with another project.

Once the risks of an innovation project are known and addressed, the innovator can proceed to establish a plan for production and marketing the new business, along with a forecast of sales and production or selling expenses. Key in the assumptions underlying these forecasts are any plans to market or promote the new product or service and any determinations of how the product will be produced for market. These plans and their resulting estimates are used to first establish a volume of sales needed to break even and then create a set of projected financial statements: profit and loss statement, cash flow statement, and balance sheet.

This phase can also be a potential stopping point for some projects. If the costs of bringing an innovation to market are high, the price charged for the product might be prohibitively high—a factor that could limit the market for the innovation or require an initial investment that is too high to attract funders. Some firms conduct extensive research and pricing analyses to determine the **price sensitivity** of purchasing the product or service. A high cost structure may create such a high breakeven point—the point at which revenues are sufficient to cover all costs of production, sales, and overhead costs—that the quantity of sales or amount of revenues may also need to be very high (perhaps higher than can be expected in the market) just to recover all costs. This consideration can be significantly influential in the implementation decision if the product or service is aimed at an area of the industry where revenues may be falling. One example is a service provided by a healthcare provider where insurance reimbursements are limited or subject to decline. Some ventures may help reduce costs in providing care, but a large up-front investment could be considered prohibitive. In such an instance, the entrepreneur may need to

**Price sensitivity**
An estimate of how much a consumer will change the quantity purchased of a good or service based on a change in price for that good or service.

reevaluate the means by which a product or service comes to market or further explore the potential volume of sales to be sure sales volume will be sufficient to offset all costs and generate a positive return for the venture.

Successfully resolving these financial and production questions takes the project to the point where management or investors can finally prioritize which projects go into full development, testing, and ultimately launch in the market. This stage is gate 3 in the phase-gate process, the point at which the venture moves from an entrepreneurial innovation to an ongoing operational management process.

## Disruptive Innovation

Much of the entrepreneurial innovation in healthcare has sought ways to earn additional income from the existing healthcare system. As this push for income from investors and healthcare business ventures continues, the actual services to address illness and injury—the essence of healthcare delivery—become less affordable. In other words, as the industry adds new technology believed to solve the challenges currently facing the US healthcare system, the costs of delivering services is continually driven upward (Hwang and Christensen 2008; Christensen, Grossman, and Hwang 2009). In some respects, this trend seems rational because the successful entrepreneur develops a business that preserves or expands revenue and income. However, when faced with the prospect that the current state of affairs in the healthcare industry must change because of its disproportionate drain on the country's gross domestic product, some entrepreneurs aim to completely change the delivery of these services and make them more affordable. In so doing, they expect to reap benefits from implementing a less complicated, and thus less expensive, product that will be more widely sought in the industry than is currently offered. Entrepreneurs who seek this type of innovation are engaged in disruptive innovation.

Disruptive innovation is a type of change in an industry that combines cost-reducing technology with alteration to the fundamental business model by which products are taken to market. Other industries have undergone such change in recent history. For example, prior to the 1970s, air travel was considered a luxury available only to the very wealthy. In some respects, healthcare is no different even today, as despite the presence of market reforms created by the Affordable Care Act, a large proportion of the US population does not have access to adequate healthcare due to the high costs of such services.

However, just as disruptive innovators such as Herb Kelleher and Southwest Airlines introduced fundamental and significant change in the delivery of air travel services, reducing the cost of air travel to the extent that it was an affordable means of transportation rather than an expensive luxury, disruptive innovation in healthcare seeks to achieve the Triple Aim of improved outcomes, reduced costs, and improved patient satisfaction.

**Technological enabler**
An advancement in the way things have been done in the past.

Disruptive innovation requires three critical elements: a **techno-logical enabler**, an innovation to the existing business model, and a value proposition (Christensen, Grossman, and Hwang 2009). The technological enabler is some advancement in the way activities have been carried out or processes have been completed in the past that streamlines or converts it to a systematic—almost assembly line–like—means of completion. Processes that require some degree of interpretation, intuition, or experience are those ripe for disruptive change. Healthcare has many such processes, some of which are deeply entrenched in routine. Examples include the manual review of medication orders by a pharmacist, and the copying of insurance cards by registration staff. As part of its innovation of air travel, Southwest Airlines simplified its passenger reservation system to eliminate seat assignments and flight reservations, significantly reducing the cost of selling plane tickets by managing the passenger boarding process. In turn, these fundamental process changes lowered the cost of air travel to the average consumer. Similar healthcare-related disruptive technological innovations are the integration of a barcode reader with a computerized provider order entry system to verify appropriateness of the medication order and the automated downloading of insurance and demographic information from an insurer database to a healthcare facility's patient accounting system. Other examples include the expansion of tools to facilitate the use of evidence-based medicine and simplifications to the rollout of genetic-based therapies for diseases such as cancer. Given the challenges of healthcare entrepreneurism, none of these promising ideas has been fully implemented.

The second critical component of disruptive innovation, innovation to the existing business model, entails a substantial change in the way services are delivered using a lower-cost technology. Again using the example of Southwest Airlines, the lower-cost approach to selling tickets and getting passengers on airplanes indicated that Southwest could be more profitable to the extent that it could keep its airplanes flying more and sitting on the ground less—a fundamental change in the operating paradigm for airlines at that time. The lowered cost and greater in-flight frequency enabled Southwest to profit from its innovation.

An important note about this example is that government regulations may prevent some changes from occurring to current business models. While Southwest did not face such hurdles with its operational changes in boarding passengers, it did face regulatory hurdles that dictated what airports it could directly connect with. For decades, Southwest could not fly directly from Dallas Love Field airport to airports beyond cities in the states bordering Texas. That said, Southwest's model was so innovative that it was profitable despite this limitation. Considering the impact of regulatory limitations in changing healthcare-related processes as well is a necessary part of the innovation process. In some cases, the entrepreneur may need to seek amendment to such regulations to advance a disruptive innovation.

Finally, the **value proposition**—the most important of the three critical elements of disruptive innovation—is significant to the entrepreneur in that the proposed change may present a greater benefit to the consumer than that currently available in the market. The proposed innovation must be an improvement in terms of perceived utility to the consumer for the same or a lower price to be attractive and ultimately successful in the marketplace. Southwest Airlines faced a significant opportunity in the value proposition for air travel compared to other means of personal transportation, such as bus or automobile transportation. When Southwest succeeded in bringing its new model of air travel to market, the value proposition was attractive to consumers who were willing to pay the price charged by Southwest to take a trip by airplane rather than take the time and trouble to drive the same distance.

**Value proposition**
A belief that the proposed change will present benefits to the consumer.

Healthcare faces a slightly different challenge in presenting a value proposition. Southwest Airlines presented an attractive value proposition because the distance to be traveled and the cost of resources to cover that distance were known in advance. Southwest was able to predict costs and sell tickets at a profitable rate. The same may not be true in all aspects of healthcare, as the costs of a surgery or procedure may not be known until the procedure is performed and other health-related conditions or complications are accounted for. This factor alone can represent an opportunity to improve the consumer's value proposition for healthcare if a consumer can find an affordable source of care that does not pose a significant risk in terms of additional price.

Ventures that can streamline processes and lower costs or make them more predictable to both the seller and the consumer represent an improvement to the current value proposition in healthcare. One example is the emergence of primary care clinics in retail pharmacy and department stores. These types of services present an enhanced value proposition for basic healthcare services, giving a predictable price for a prospectively set array of services. While some healthcare needs exceed the capabilities of such a clinic, the majority of routine care can be delivered within the average consumer's financial means in a setting that is familiar to him. Another example of disruptive innovation in healthcare services is the advent of cardiac angioplasty, which was seen as a lower-cost intervention for partially occluded arteries in the heart. Prior to this innovation, patients faced the prospect of open-heart surgery and a long—and expensive—convalescence. Angioplasty altered the landscape for that healthcare need to a largely outpatient and low-cost procedure with a markedly shorter time for recovery.

The essence of disruptive innovation in healthcare is that it brings a new technological advancement (e.g., the cardiac stent) while simultaneously modifying existing processes (inserting the stent into the heart artery via a guide wire rather than by opening the artery), thereby addressing a need in the marketplace (demand for a lower-cost intervention for partially blocked cardiac arteries). The healthcare industry has heavily entrenched interests in maintaining current ways of delivering care through high-cost hospitals and expensive medical specialists, because it is profitable for those parties that sell current technology. The deep entrenchment of those interests creates a significant opportunity for the entrepreneur who can identify a new technology or process, integrate it into a new business model, and do so in a way that brings improved value to the consumer.

## Summary

Healthcare organizations, ranging from academic medical centers to safety-net hospital systems to large multispecialty physician groups, realize that the landscape is changing so fast that traditional improvement approaches are not keeping pace. Recent developments, including new consumer digital technology, financial incentives via accountable care organizations, and access to large health data sets, are enhancing the opportunity for innovation (Jain and Tsang 2014). Whatever the approach to generating, screening, and implementing new ideas at hospitals, health systems, or other organizations, the purpose of innovation remains the same: "It is generating a core competency inside your organization to generate new care models, new service lines, new business models that prepare you for the future," according to John Gallagher, practice leader for innovation at Simpler Consulting, a division of Truven Health Analytics, who works with health systems to create specialized innovation teams (quoted in Raths 2015).

## Discussion Questions

1. Name and explain several major challenges facing the US healthcare delivery system.
2. What role can be played by entrepreneurship and innovation in solving many of the challenges encountered in healthcare delivery today?

3. Name and explain the most important factors to creating entrepreneurial opportunities in the healthcare sector of the US economy.
4. Explain the role of innovation in the delivery of healthcare services in the United States.

# References

Ackerly, D., A. Valverde, L. Diener, K. Dossary, and K. Schulman. 2009. "Fueling Innovation in Medical Devices (and Beyond): Venture Capital in Health Care." *Health Affairs* 28 (1): 68–75.

Asoh, D. A., P. A. Rivers, K. J. McCleary, and P. Savela. 2005. "Entrepreneurial Propensity in Health Care: Models and Propositions for Empirical Research." *Health Care Management Review* 30 (3): 212–19.

Audia, P. G., and C. I. Rider. 2005. "A Garage and an Idea: What More Does an Entrepreneur Need?" *California Management Review*. Accessed November 26, 2016. http://mba.tuck.dartmouth.edu/pages/faculty/pino.audia/docs/garage%20myth%20CMR.pdf.

Center for Responsive Politics. 2016. "Lobbying Spending Database." Accessed December 26. www.opensecrets.org/lobby/top.php?showYear=2015&indexType=s.

Christensen, C. M., J. Grossman, and J. Hwang. 2009. *The Innovator's Prescription: A Disruptive Solution for Health Care*. New York: McGraw-Hill.

Drucker, P. F. 1993. *Innovation and Entrepreneurship*. New York: Harper.

Garrety, K., I. McLoughlin, and G. Zelle. 2014. "Disruptive Innovation in Health Care: Business Models, Moral Orders and Electronic Records." *Social Policy and Society* 13: 579–92.

Guo, K. L. 2003. "Applying Entrepreneurship to Health Care Organizations." *New England Journal of Entrepreneurship* 6 (1): 45–53.

Herzlinger, R. E. 2006. "Why Innovation in Health Care Is So Hard." *Harvard Business Review*. Published May. https://hbr.org/2006/05/why-innovation-in-health-care-is-so-hard.

Hwang, J., and C. M. Christensen. 2008. "Disruptive Innovation in Health Care Delivery: A Framework for Business-Model Innovation." *Health Affairs* 27 (5): 1329–35.

Jain, S. H., and T. Tsang. 2014. "Health Care Becomes Entrepreneurial (Finally)." *Harvard Business Review*. Published May 26. https://hbr.org/2014/05/health-care-becomes-entrepreneurial-finally/.

Kuratko, D., and R. Hodgetts. 1998. *Entrepreneurship: A Contemporary Approach*. Fort Worth, TX: Dryden.

Lamantia, J. 2015. "Oscar's Losses Are Huge—and Investors Don't Care; How One Insurance Startup with Only 40,000 Members Is Worth $1.5 Billion." *Crain's New York Business* 31 (August 10): 4.

Martin, R. L. 2011. "The Innovation Catalysts." *Harvard Business Review.* Published June. https://hbr.org/2011/06/the-innovation-catalysts.

McCreary, L. 2010. "Kaiser Permanente's Innovation on the Front Lines." *Harvard Business Review.* Published September. https://hbr.org/2010/09/kaiser-permanentes-innovation-on-the-front-lines.

Meyers, A. 2015. "Health Entrepreneurship on the Rise." *Modern Healthcare.* Published February 21. www.modernhealthcare.com/article/20150221/MAGAZINE/302219978.

PricewaterhouseCoopers. 2000. *Healthcast 2010: Report on the Future of the Health Care Industry.* New York: PricewaterhouseCoopers.

Raths, D. 2015. "Does Your Health System Need an Innovation Center?" *Healthcare Informatics.* Published December 8. www.healthcare-informatics.com/blogs/david-raths/does-your-health-system-need-innovation-center.

Roggenkamp, S. D., and K. R. White. 1998. "Four Nurse Entrepreneurs: What Motivated Them to Start Their Own Business." *Health Care Management Review* 23 (3): 67–75.

Schumpeter, J. A. 1936. *The Theory of Economic Development*, 2nd ed. Cambridge, MA: Harvard University Press.

Timmons, J. A. 1989. *The Entrepreneurial Mind.* Andover, MA: Brick House.

# THE DEVELOPMENT OF TRUST IN HEALTHCARE ORGANIZATIONS

Tina Marie Evans

"I'm not upset that you lied to me. I'm upset that from now on I can't believe you."

—Friedrich Wilhelm Nietzsche

## Learning Objectives

After completing this chapter, the reader should be able to

- explain the significance of trust in manager–employee relationships,
- explain the significance of trust in healthcare provider–patient relationships,
- describe ways trust can be built,
- describe how trust can be lost,
- explain the role of communication in trust, and
- articulate the steps that can be taken to reclaim lost trust.

## Key Terms and Concepts

- Authentic
- Bonding
- Breach of trust
- Integrity
- Involuntary trust

- Legacy
- Mission statement
- Sociopathy
- Trust

## Introduction

From a humanistic perspective, healthcare systems are built on the unique personal qualities of a wide variety of people. Because the set of relationships at play is complex, some of the most difficult challenges for healthcare managers are rooted in relationship-based trust issues. If your employees do not trust you, why would they choose to follow you? People tend to be suspicious of those in leadership roles, whether inside or outside of healthcare settings. The interactions between healthcare managers and other personnel either go smoothly or go so roughly that they tear apart the very fiber of an organization. Earning trust is a critical aspect of healthcare management, as it can be viewed as the glue that holds the hospital or health system together. On the other hand, a lack of trust can cause innumerable problems, all of which take away from the mission and purpose of the work.

Dye (2000, 111) suggests leaders pause to think about how unimaginable these daily activities would be without **trust:**

**Trust**
A feeling that connotes honesty and reliability.

> Imagine convincing people whom you do not trust and who do not trust you to cooperate. Imagine sharing information with them. Imaging collaborating with them. Imagine asking them for help. If you can imagine any of these scenarios without feeling paranoid, doubtful, exhausted, desperate, exasperated, and doomed, then I salute you; please skip to the next chapter. If you cannot, please keep reading.

Competency alone does not build the trusting relations that all healthcare managers should strive for. Generally, either people trust you or they don't. This chapter defines trust and its importance to leadership in healthcare.

## What Is Trust, and Why Is It Important?

*Trust* is defined in the online Merriam-Webster Collegiate Dictionary (2016) as the "assured reliance on the character, ability, strength, or truth of someone or something." In general, trust is a relational phenomenon whereby a person or an entity is honest, reliable, and of good intention. It may be found in oneself, interrelationally between two or more people, between people and organizations, or between people and events. In its simplest form, trust is a psychological state. To trust another person is a personal choice made on the basis of the expectation or belief that the other person or entity will or will not act a certain way in a given situation. This expectation is usually held to be correct over time. If the expectation is violated by a **breach of trust**, disappointment and negativity often result (Gilson 2003). Therefore, trust carries an inherent level of risk for individuals because of the unavoidable level of uncertainty over another's motives, intentions, and actions.

**Breach of trust**
Failure to act in a way that is expected based on confidence in and reliance on the actor.

# The Benefits of Earning Trust

Many benefits accrue from maintaining trust in organizations. Managers who confidently trust their staff are more self-assured, more open and honest, more willing to take risks, less resistant to change, and more inclined to act in a trustworthy manner themselves than are managers who lack trust in their direct reports. From both sides, trust is an empowering state. Consider the professional bonding that trust allows to take place in a working environment. This **bonding** builds a sense of community among the employees, who over time come to care about each other and about the work they share. Such a positive dynamic is comfortable and comforting, and it is sought by many employees.

**Bonding**
The building of a sense of community among employees.

Similarly, having employees who rely on your honesty is rewarding as well. Information sharing and collaboration activities tend to be productive and positive when employees trust that they will be given fair credit for their contributions and ideas and that sensitive pieces of information shared will be kept in strict confidence by the manager. Such trusting and open environments provide an ideal context for brainstorming innovative ideas as well as resolving conflicts effectively. In times of difficulty when many options are under consideration, managers who have earned the trust of their employees are in an enhanced position to discuss the options and persuade some to change their mind, as trust allows others to be influenced. Without trust, employees may not consider the manager's options, proposals, or resolutions—even if they are in the best interest of the overall organization.

Distance, whether physically real or perceived by the employees, is a major factor in the earning of trust. The greater the distance between the manager and the employees, the more room for interpretation—and misinterpretation—and the greater the chance that the manager is not trusted. Having an office far away from those being supervised is not an optimal situation. Employees need to see and interact with the manager. An interactive, collegial environment characterized by a positive, friendly managerial presence facilitates the day-to-day work of the organization.

As trust is built, the questioning of motives and intentions in situations lessens over time. If employees (or the manager) are constantly compelled to question the motives and intentions of others, progress comes to a halt as they take the time to consider the level of risk involved in each situation.

In addition, a manager's trust in her employees fosters an environment in which she may delegate appropriate tasks to them. Furthermore, employees who trust their managers are inclined to work diligently for the good of the organization and may choose to take on additional responsibilities. This response is even more common when the manager facilitates a trusting environment in which others are comfortable knowing that honest mistakes are treated as learning opportunities rather than seen as a direct threat to their employment. With this understanding, employees tend to be quick to accept new or difficult tasks, as the punishment for an honest mistake is downplayed.

Trust is a central benefit to managers in their work, particularly in times of challenge, change, and organizational uncertainty. Managers who take the time to build a solid foundation of trust with their employees are poised to navigate tough situations with little resistance. On the other hand, employees who do not trust their managers are suspect of managers' motives during times of trouble and hesitate to go above and beyond if needed. Regardless of the situation, nontrusting employees often perform to the minimum level required of their positions. Trusting employees, in times of challenge, tend to exceed required levels of performance to help bring a positive result for the team and resolve the tough situation.

Truth telling is another component of trust. Autonomy in both employee and patient decision making involves consistent truth telling. Human interactions are based on the assumption of truth as the basis of trust. Therefore, patients, care providers, and managers all must be able to work from the perspective that honesty is the norm rather than the exception. The confidence that comes with this trust is central to good relationships in all categories. By virtue of their powerful administrative position, managers have the ethical responsibility of truth telling. Lying (whether intentionally or by omission) has destroyed the careers of many managers, in part because lying or omitting truthfulness leads to decreased employee performance, resentment, and retention issues. Dosick (2000) also warns that dishonesty causes a loss of integrity (discussed in depth later in the chapter) and may lead to the loss of your position. To reap the benefits of trust, honesty must be the prevailing policy. Lying and dishonesty are damaging to all relationships; just one lie can allow the foundation of a trusting relationship to crumble.

Along the same lines, one benefit of being able to trust the word and promises of others, and of instilling trust in your words and promises, is its impact on successful outcomes. Mutual trust has long been recognized as a key dimension of managerial success, as operations can only run smoothly when promises to perform are kept. Trustworthiness is an expectation in society (not just in the healthcare industry); therefore, leaders must constantly be aware of what they say and what promises they make to whom. Words and actions set the tone for interactions, and careful selection of those words and actions is critical. Managers also are cautioned that in some situations, silence may be viewed as agreement, as staff may trust that silence is consent in the absence of any other indicators about the manager's position on a matter. As leaders, you must have the courage to speak your thoughts and set the record straight, whether verbally or by written communication. Be clear about where you stand in each situation, and do not give others the opportunity to make assumptions.

# Developing Trust at the Managerial Level

Trust does not occur automatically or emerge overnight; it takes active attention and consistent dedication to allow trust to build over time. Once it is built, it must be carefully cultivated, protected, and maintained. Given that people tend to harbor natural suspicions of those in leadership positions, managers must acknowledge that they start out with the burden to prove they are trustworthy. Recognizing this natural suspicion and then acting accordingly helps you earn the trust of your employees over time. This section presents seven approaches for trust building in organizations; the next section shares seven points of caution regarding how trust can be lost. First, we focus on the process of trust building. Managers seeking to actively build trust should take the following measures.

## Be Honest and Authentic

The more managers can be viewed as **authentic** people who take the time to be available to their colleagues and staff, the greater is the difficulty to view them with suspicion. Achieving authenticity takes work, but it is a worthwhile effort for becoming a high-performing manager.

**Authentic**
Demonstrating genuine characteristics to others at all times, thereby showing worthiness of their trust.

Senior leaders frequently talk about "engaging the hearts and minds of employees and physicians," but that ability requires individuals to "first be connected to the heart and the mind of the leader" (Dye and Garman 2015, 55). Outwardly demonstrating that you honestly care about connecting authentically with those around you and caring about their work is a cornerstone of good leadership. Good leaders are not afraid to let their employees know they care. High-performing managers take steps to instill confidence that staff can do their jobs knowing their leader is competent to run the organization effectively. By putting their staff members' minds at ease that all is well and they are working for a competent and capable leader, a manager allows staff to focus on the task at hand rather than be distracted by questions about the leader's abilities.

## Be Open

In healthcare organizations, environments characterized by open and candid interactions foster the development of trust. Managers should promote an environment in which all are encouraged to speak freely and honestly while sharing ideas and concerns. Employees should not have to worry about repercussions resulting from their interactions. If they make positive contributions, the manager should thank them for these contributions and for taking the initiative to present their ideas or concerns for consideration.

When a manager disseminates information, he should do so in a timely, effective manner depending on the situation (e.g., verbally in a meeting, individually in private, via e-mail). He should accurately share news and findings without holding back key information. Hiding information is detrimental to maintaining or building trust. Especially in cases of unwelcome news, the manager should not be afraid to share the information in a tactful way. Allowing employees to fill in missing information by talking among themselves about what may be happening behind the scenes perpetuates an environment of secrecy.

### Be Reliable and Consistent

Predictability and consistency in a leader are traits that contribute to the trust-building effort. Being reliable and consistent means doing what you say you will do. Over time, employees' confidence grows with the knowledge that the manager is true to his word and can be trusted.

A manager who demonstrates inconsistent behavior, on the other hand, such as giving conflicting messages, begs employees to view her as erratic and therefore untrustworthy. Unpredictability creates a stressful and unpleasant work environment for staff.

Employees often associate temperament with reliability and consistency. A manager who acts friendly and outgoing one day then moody and down-spirited the next day negatively affects those around her (Dye 2000). A calm demeanor and positive attitude around employees help staff be at ease under trying circumstances.

### Be Accessible

The development of trust is facilitated when managers are open with and available to their employees. This accessibility allows confidence to develop among personnel and leads to the free sharing of thoughts and feelings. Efforts to greet employees each morning as a matter of common courtesy and respect, for example, help establish a conception of the manager as approachable and reasonable. Another tactic to demonstrate accessibility is to allow some room on meeting agendas for raising concerns and sharing new ideas. This space can be listed as the last agenda item to ensure that all other important business is handled first; the key is to make sure time is devoted to this type of discussion. Think about how many good ideas are not shared because of strictly controlled meeting agendas that do not allow for open discussions.

### Lead by Example

It is no secret that for those in management positions, others are watching. A manager's goal should not be to please everyone around him but to accomplish the goals he has set out to accomplish. If the manager's leadership values are clear, those around him know exactly what he stands for. Will he step in and help when needed? In times of stress or crisis, does he willingly do his part to resolve it? Setting a good example as a hard worker communicates to staff that the manager can be trusted because they will see he is dedicated to success and unafraid to participate in resolutions (Dye and Garman 2015).

### Honor Your Promises

As an extension of reliability, honoring promises is vital to building trust. If a manager makes a promise, she must follow through and fulfill it. If she absolutely cannot keep the stated promise, she must explain to the employee or group (face-to-face) why she cannot fulfill it. She needs to be clear and honest in her explanation, taking care not to diminish the significance of the promise.

A manager should never promise more than she can deliver with certainty in the stated time frame. Any uncertainty about the situation should be raised with others to clarify concerns, doubts, risks, and confounding variables. Good managers avoid making promises they cannot meet. They do not feel compelled to manage by constantly making promises to others. Instead, they understand that not promising or committing to an action or a result that may not be deliverable is sometimes appropriate. In short, making a promise means doing everything one can to hold oneself accountable to one's word.

### Drive Out Fear

In his book *Beyond the Wall of Resistance*, Rick Maurer (1996) states that the opposite of trust is fear and theorizes that a lack of trust sparks a pattern of fear. This suggestion is one that all managers should take a moment to appreciate. Distrust and fear can escalate among employees to feelings of negativity, anxiety, and resistance to change.

Maurer (1996) explains that building the support needed for organizational change is difficult, if not impossible, without trust. If employees are fearful and anxious, they are likely to either fight or lie low; neither of these responses moves the organization forward to make the changes needed to be successful.

## How Not to Develop Trust

Just as some leadership behaviors engender trust, others destroy it. To avoid the latter types of behaviors, awareness is necessary for all healthcare managers. In particular, they should not adopt or continue to manage using the following traits.

### Be Unavailable

Some managers are happy to be left alone and to stay in their office, perhaps hoping to avoid interactions because they are uncomfortable interacting with others, or because the sheer amount of time required to perform the needed tasks of the job is overwhelming. A manager whose leadership style is reserved should recognize that he will struggle to earn his employees' trust. They need to see and interact with him on a regular basis to develop expectations of consistency, reliability, and other trust-building attributes.

### Fail to Demonstrate Concern

Managerially speaking, *having* concern for employees differs greatly from *showing* concern for them. The first is a passive state, and the second is an active state. Some managers may meet with and engage their employees on a regular basis but fail to convey genuine concern about the challenges employees face. Managers and staff are all on the same team. Exhibiting concern conveys a true sense of team engagement that builds trust over time by allowing the employees to see that the manager does indeed care about what is happening (Dye and Garman 2015).

### Fail to Lead by Example

Failing to lead by example is among the most damaging habits a manager can demonstrate. A manager who is viewed as hypocritical, tyrannical, disengaged, or full of self-importance sets herself up for struggles over trustworthiness. Managers should always act as they expect their employees to act in the workplace—with no exceptions. As the leader, the manager must set the desired image and standard.

### Be Inconsistent and Fail to Follow Through

Not following up with staff can be perceived as callous or malicious, even if this is not the manager's intent. If the manager says he will get an employee the answer to a question or send a staff member an informational file by the end of the week, he needs to do so. Dye and Garman (2015, 57) note that failing to follow up is often the result of "an over-willingness to make promises without considering what it will take to make good on them." Yet some managers have not developed their organizational skills to the level where they can accurately keep track of what they stated they would do for whom. Most often, people can forgive this type of error if it is a one-time occurrence. If it becomes habitual, however, trust can be quickly eroded.

### Give Credit to or Blame the Wrong Person

Healthcare managers erode trust when they give credit to an undeserving staff member for success or blame the wrong person for a failure. Whether contributions are positive or negative, managers should take the time to understand who the true contributors are in a given situation, and they should be especially cautious in rushed, heated, or otherwise stressful situations. Good leaders do not guess—they verify the name of each contributor and thank each for his or her contribution to a successful project.

Managers should also be alert for slips of the tongue, as when describing the work of their employees by saying "I" when the group should be acknowledged with gratitude in public. Failing to give appropriate credit may leave those affected with the feeling that the hard work is simply not worth it, which damages productivity (Dye and Garman 2015).

Blaming the wrong person can carry even more severe implications because blame is damaging to an individual's professional reputation, and the manager who blames the wrong person damages her own reputation as well. When a leader misplaces blame, she must sincerely apologize for any such error in person to the employee.

## *Breach Confidentiality*

In the managerial role, great care must be taken to protect a vast amount of information, including (but not limited to) employee relations, disciplinary actions, impending layoffs or reductions in the workforce, employee misconduct, and terminations. Even in cases where the disclosure of such sensitive types of information may not be illegal, it is counterproductive, and the manager who does so will damage his image in the eyes of his employees. In addition to making a concerted effort to protect this information, managers must have in place a clear, up-to-date confidentiality policy for employees to follow. If the policy is violated, the manager must be consistent in disciplining those in violation of it by invoking the stated procedures.

## *Lie*

Managers have been known to lie to their subordinates. In the absence of **sociopathy**, lying in the workplace typically reflects attempts to avoid tough situations and issues, such as the need to break bad news to one or more employees. Lying is frowned upon, even at the level of simple white lies, such as not answering a difficult question truthfully or not telling an employee why he was not promoted.

**Sociopathy**
Antisocial behavior characterized by a lack of a sense of moral responsibility and lack of good conscience.

Important to note here is that lying is viewed differently from withholding information. Healthcare managers are often privy to levels of information that cannot be freely shared with all employees for a variety of reasons. In situations where a manager is questioned about information that cannot be shared, she should simply state that it is not possible to disclose information about the topic, rather than lying about it.

Overall, if employees are unable to trust their manager, many facets of productivity falter. Communication and collaboration suffer. Additionally, turnover increases while morale decreases. Managers who are aware of these positive and negative behaviors can make their organization's environment a place of trust, honesty, innovation, and creativity, and subsequently one that achieves high-quality outcomes.

## Developing Trust in the Provider–Patient Relationship

Although this chapter is mostly concerned with trust between leaders and staff or others in the organization, managers should also have a strong awareness of the trust dynamic in the healthcare provider–patient relationship, which is central to the successful provision of healthcare services. This provider–patient interaction is an important two-way relationship in which one offers care and services to the other, who freely and willingly accepts them. The process of seeking healthcare involves a certain level of vulnerability, as a power imbalance is inherent between those who have the knowledge to provide the care and those who are in the position of need.

The level of trust that underlies this relationship can have a positive impact on the patient, as the peace of mind that comes from a trusting situation can facilitate healing. As care is provided, a trusting provider–patient relationship eases the communication process between the parties and prompts the disclosure of necessary information from the patient, which only improves the care provided.

Healthcare providers are expected to show an impartial concern for all patients' overall well-being regardless of the specific situation, including any funding mechanisms that may affect this fiduciary relationship. This expectation is especially important in cases where a patient is unable to speak or make decisions on his own behalf. In emergency situations, a form of **involuntary trust** must quickly form in light of the critical nature of emergency care, which heightens the expectation placed on the providers. Involuntary trust is viewed by some as a form of dependency, yet it is protected by codes of ethics established by professional organizations as well as ethical codes promulgated by the healthcare organization. Vulnerable patients must be protected from exploitation of trust, as the power differential is remarkable in certain situations.

The healthcare manager's role is an important one, wherein he must state the expectations, remind providers of those expectations, and monitor activities for all dimensions of ethical correctness. To effectively manage the patient–provider trust dynamic, leaders must understand how that trust develops. Gopichandran and Chetlapalli (2013) conducted a study that used patient interviews to evaluate the key dimensions of trust in patients' healthcare providers. The authors concluded that the most pertinent dimensions of trust building in this relationship were the following:

**Involuntary trust**
A default state of trust that is created between two parties in light of a power imbalance and the necessity of dependency of one party on the other party for care.

- Perceived competence
- Assurance of treatment irrespective of ability to pay or time of day
- Patient's willingness to accept potential drawbacks in healthcare
- Patient's loyalty to the physician
- Patient's respect for the physician

The patient's *perceived* comfort level with the physician and healthcare facility, the personal involvement (or its absence) of the physician with the patient, the behavior and approach of the physician, prevailing economic factors, and health awareness were also identified as dimensions that determine the level of trust in healthcare providers.

Furthermore, Hall and colleagues (2001) describe fidelity, competence, honesty, confidentiality, and global trust as key aspects of trust in the provider–patient relationship. From the author's experience, fidelity can be described as respect for the patient's agency or autonomy as a person and the ability to keep the patient's welfare in mind during all interactions and at all stages of care provision. Competence in diagnosis and treatment has also been emphasized as essential for the building of trust. Finally, Gopichandran and Chetlapalli (2013) note that being honest, acting in a transparent manner, and maintaining confidentiality can be considered aspects of trust building.

Managers can aid in clinicians' efforts to enhance the provider–patient relationship by sharing these insights about involuntary trust and overall trust building with physicians, nurses, and ancillary personnel to improve their awareness toward solidifying trust.

## Integrity in Leadership

Morrison (2011) explains that although managers do not directly provide healthcare services, conduct research, or design technologies used in the clinical setting, they are nonetheless critical to the success of all those functions because they control and set the tone for the environment in which each takes place. In addition to obtaining a working knowledge of system functions, finance, human resources management, and leadership, both healthcare managers and providers must develop a clear understanding of personal and professional ethics and use this understanding as the basis on which to build a trusting relationship with patients, employees, the organization, and the larger community. This awareness is the essence of **integrity**.

Trust and integrity in healthcare may seem like simplistic principles, but ethical situations that challenge a manager's and employees' ability to

**Integrity**
The consistent demonstration of honesty and strong moral principles.

respect autonomy are common in today's healthcare environment. The organization and the entire community count on managers to rise to these challenges and act to preserve the rights of all in the situations they encounter. At a minimum, managers should review the organization's mission statements periodically, aim their continuing education efforts toward ethical practice and the importance of trust, and observe and evaluate employees regularly in terms of the dimensions of integrity—honesty, correctness in values, consistency in ethical behavior as defined by professional codes, and demonstration of strong moral character, among many others.

Having insight on how policies and procedures are perceived by others gives the manager additional information with which to lead and fosters the building of trust with employees. A significant responsibility of managers is to create, and orient staff to, a climate that is consistent with the mission and values of the organization and with the expectations of the employees and patients. As a matter of integrity, managers must educate and keep themselves updated on the discipline of ethics so that the work climate is well understood by all and a clear process is in place to resolve any ethical situations that arise. In terms of fairness, the leader with integrity ensures that all staff members are aware of what is expected of them in their positions and communicates any changes to those expectations in a timely manner (Healey and Marchese 2012). This aspect of integrity reflects the openness component of trust discussed earlier in this chapter.

Integrity and trust also come into play when dealing with employee discipline. Boyle and colleagues (2001) explain how formal discipline must be consistent from case to case to preserve perceptions of integrity and to keep employee morale intact. If a manager consistently treats all his employees in a fair way, they are likely to treat each other fairly. But if inequity is perceived (whether or not it is real), the atmosphere in the workplace deteriorates.

Managers must also ensure that the working environment is free of discrimination and harassment. If violations of stated policies occur, suitable sanctions should be applied to those in violation and these actions documented. Employees take the policies and procedures only as seriously as they see the manager taking them, so the manager must publicly acknowledge and uphold them. Each decision made is a building block of the manager's reputation, so acting with integrity toward all is a daily necessity.

**Legacy**
The qualities and values that one will be remembered for in one's work.

The demands of the administrative role can make these tasks challenging, but by paying consistent attention to managerial choices—owning them—and being aware of the consequent responsibility for them, managers are on their way to becoming leaders of integrity. Gilbert (2007) discusses personal integrity as a part of one's **legacy**, mindfulness, and choice.

Employees as well as superiors observe what you do (and, in some cases, fail to do), and Gilbert's research is clear that they will form an opinion on the basis of these observations. Managers are advised to think about integrity as part of their training to help develop their moral senses, evaluate biases, and establish a set of integrity-based values. The choices made as managers must be consistent with their personal values. If they are not, these leaders will have a hard time finding personal peace.

Managers who realize they have failed to make the best possible decision must use that situation as a learning opportunity to avoid making the same error in the future and perhaps create a good outcome out of that negative encounter. What moral lesson can be found in that experience? Another helpful activity is to think of one's managerial career as a path that allows one to make a difference in others' lives, not just an obligation to fulfill on a daily basis. A manager's legacy of integrity is built step by step, slowly over time (Healey and Marchese 2012). How do you want your supervisors and employees to remember you and your work?

## Dangers of Losing or Not Gaining Trust

We have discussed the benefits of developing a trusting environment as a manager and, in the process, have touched on some corresponding dangers of losing or failing to maintain that trust. But what is the real cost of losing trust in a healthcare organization? Simon (2002, 18), in his study of the impact on an organization's bottom line of failing to lead by example, explains that "staffers may be less engaged in their work, less receptive to new ideas, and less willing to follow the leader on the next offensive." If employees see an inconsistency in what managers say and do, a chain of events commences that reflects a deflation of trust, commitment, and willingness to achieve beyond expectations. At a minimum, these effects lead to lowered employee satisfaction, increased employee turnover, and decreased organizational profitability. Simons (2002, 19) summarizes as follows: "The notion that behavioral integrity is important should be common sense: Align your words and actions in a way employees see. Keep your promises."

Among the most dangerous ramifications of losing trust, however, is a manager's inability to see an integrity problem in herself. Naturally, managers want to see themselves as trusting, ethical, and consistent, but often they lack these characteristics. Whether a manager is just learning about leadership and supervision or is a seasoned professional, a careful periodic self-assessment of her behavioral integrity is worth the time given the high cost of this problem.

## The Role of Communication in Building Trust

Communication is described by Belasen, Eisenberg, and Huppertz (2016, 11) as a "vibrant thread that ties together employee vitality, clarity of direction and purpose, and results and progress." Their work affirms that effective leaders are skilled at using communication to achieve the goals of the organization, but communication must be used honestly and strategically. An overabundance of communication does not guarantee employees will be happy and engaged in their work. In fact, overcommunicating may be as destructive as undercommunicating.

However, the larger caution is with undercommunicating, which can lead to distrust, uncertainty, low morale, and a lack of alignment. What types of information need to be shared with employees? How much should be shared? How often should the communications take place? What is the best way to disseminate the information? Having well-considered answers for all these questions is vital to properly assessing communication methods and frequency.

Effective managers are talented communicators because they ensure that all who need to receive information will indeed receive and understand it. Communication is time intensive, and shortcuts may be tempting; however, the best possible method for both the leader and followers must be sought and used. Methods of communication vary, and that fact can be advantageous. The key is to match the best method to the individual situation, taking into consideration whether the manager can verify that the message was received as intended.

Dye and Garman (2015, 46) note that highly effective managers take the communication process one step further: "Beyond simply ensuring that the message is heard, they will ensure that the message is discussed. For example, they might instruct managers to explicitly incorporate discussion into their next staff meeting and then report back on what was discussed." Such cascading of communication can help ensure that key messages are accurately received.

Another often-forgotten communication in managerial practice is "thank you." This message not only honors and openly communicates the worth of the employees but also saves the manager time and trouble in dealing with low morale or, perhaps worse, constant recruitment and rehiring (Healey and Marchese 2012). Rewards, whether a verbal "thank you" or a tangible offering such as providing lunch, play a reciprocal role in developing trust and sustaining good performance.

Healthcare organizations can maximize the benefits of communication and collaboration by structuring operations in a format that supports teamwork, with specific guidelines that ensure timely, effective, open, and honest communication. Over time, these guidelines become intuitive pathways for healthcare providers to follow, and errors are likely to decrease as communication increases (Healey and Evans 2014).

Given the role of mission statements as guides for healthcare organizations, these statements can be viewed as communications of the promises that will be kept to others who seek medical care at the facility. Many organizational **mission statements** communicate a passion for high-quality service and ethical behavior. Managers must take the time to periodically review the mission statement and consider whether such a statement remains appropriate over time. Furthermore, they must communicate this information to employees, ensuring that their staff understand the mission and how this promise to those who seek care at the facility is fulfilled. Communicating that honesty is one way managers help create a working environment that promotes truth.

**Mission statement**
A formal document to explain an organization's core goals and values.

## Repairing Lost Trust

Think about some of the personal relationships in your life. How difficult are these relationships to manage when trust is lost because of dishonesty or deceit? Trust in others is fragile. Building the type of trusting relationship needed in a successful healthcare organization may take weeks, months, or years, but just one instance of mishandling can cause it permanent damage. Correct actions and dutiful protection of a trusting environment are critical, but sometimes even the most diligent manager destroys hard-earned trust in an instant. Following are recommendations for mending trust once it is lost.

- *Be patient.* Acknowledge that rebuilding trust is a process that takes a long time. Some employees will not respond to your efforts immediately, and a quick positive response is unreasonable. To insist that they trust only undermines your leadership. Give them time.

- *Admit your error.* Part of rebuilding trust is taking responsibility for what happened. Own up to the error in communications with those who were affected. Describe your mistake, what lesson(s) you have taken away from it, and what you intend to do differently in the future. If the employees feel you are withholding relevant information about the issue, their trust will remain impaired. Make your confession of the error in a sincere spirit, and give your commitment that it will not happen again.

- *Apologize.* The words "I'm sorry" go further than people often think they will in difficult situations. Most employees simply want, and are waiting, to hear these words from you. Give them an apology as a step toward healing, and explain that if you could go back and change the course of your action, you certainly would.

- *Be truthful about the situation.* Even if the truth is unpleasant, it must be communicated. In a face-to-face meeting, provide appropriate details about the message and talk openly about the situation. Then share your ideas and vision for the road to success, and solicit employees'. Honesty is one of the fastest methods of rebuilding trust.

- *Do not be afraid to appear vulnerable.* You are human, and you will make mistakes. Acknowledge your humanity, and be transparent about how you feel. Managers who are defensive about what they did wrong do not receive the trust of those around them. Employees are much more forgiving of managers who take personal responsibility for failures than of those who do not. Avoid defending your error, though doing so may seem natural.

- *Listen.* For the employee, the breach of trust may have caused anger, hurt feelings, or another negative response. Be present with those who were harmed, and hear their feelings out. Do not interrupt; just listen. Let them express their thoughts and feelings—this exercise is a healthy part of healing. To get such feelings out and be heard is important for those who have been harmed or deceived, and your allowance of it communicates that you genuinely care. Listening sounds easy, but it can be difficult in this type of situation. You may not like what you hear, but when the fault is yours, you must put distress aside.

- *Request employee feedback.* Ask staff for recommendations on resolving the situation. They may have helpful suggestions, and again, your inquiry communicates that you sincerely care about getting relations back on the right track. What would they prefer that you do differently? What are their concerns going forward? Even if their feedback is negative or harsh, act professionally and have the grace to receive their feedback with an open mind. If they have a good suggestion, implement it, and be sure to give credit to the person who generated the suggestion.

To succeed at regaining trust, you must persevere, practice patience, and consistently work at the rebuilding process. Set a higher standard for yourself than you demonstrated in the past, and commit to achieving that standard for the good of the team. Effective leadership is impossible without having trusting relationships with your employees. If you lack trust, you lack followers. And without followers, you are not a leader.

Johnson (2009) recommends identifying role models in trustworthiness. Sometimes considered mentors, these role models can serve as sounding boards, advisers, ethical guides, and living examples of how to act and not act when situations become challenging. Another recommendation is to read and reflect on the actions of well-known leaders and to evaluate case studies that have a moral dimension to help develop trust skills and prepare for integrity-based decision making.

## Summary

Trust has a constant impact on each portion of one's daily work. It surrounds and affects the quality of every relationship, every communication, every group project, and every initiative a manager oversees. It affects the quality of each moment and carries the power to change the trajectory and outcome of each future moment of a career.

Managers are encouraged to spend the time to get to know their employees; evaluate risk carefully in terms of trust relationships; work to build and maintain trust; and, when needed, not delay in taking the steps to repair lost trust.

## Discussion Questions

1. Why is trust important?
2. How can trust influence the patient–provider relationship?
3. What are some specific ways trust can be built in organizations?
4. How is trust eroded and destroyed in organizations?
5. What are the main benefits of having trust in a manager?
6. Once trust is lost, what specific steps can be taken to rebuild it?

## References

Belasen, A. T., B. Eisenberg, and J. W. Huppertz. 2016. *Mastering Leadership: A Vital Resource for Health Care Organizations.* Burlington, MA: Jones & Bartlett Learning.

Boyle, P., E. R. DuBose, S. J. Ellingson, D. E. Guinn, and D. B. McCurdy. 2001. *Organizational Ethics in Health Care: Principles, Cases and Practical Solutions.* San Francisco: Jossey-Bass.

Dosick, R. W. 2000. *The Business Bible: Ten Commandments for Creating an Ethical Workplace.* Woodstock, VT: Jewish Lights.

Dye, C. F. 2000. *Leadership in Healthcare: Values at the Top.* Chicago: Health Administration Press.

Dye, C. F., and A. N. Garman. 2015. *Exceptional Leadership: 16 Critical Competencies for Healthcare Executives.* Chicago: Health Administration Press.

Gilbert, J. A. 2007. *Strengthening Ethical Wisdom: Tools for Transforming Your Healthcare Organization.* Chicago: Health Administration Press.

Gilson, L. 2003. "Trust and the Development of Health Care as a Social Institution." *Social Science Medicine* 56 (7): 1453–68.

Gopichandran, V., and S. K. Chetlapalli. 2013. "Dimensions and Determinants of Trust in Health Care in Resource Poor Settings—a Qualitative Exploration." *PLoS ONE.* Published July 16. http://journals.plos.org/plosone/article?id=10.1371/journal.pone.0069170.

Hall, M. A., E. Dugan, B. Zheng, and A. K. Mishra. 2001. "Trust in Physicians and Medical Institutions: What Is It, Can It Be Measured, and Does It Matter?" *Milbank Quarterly* 79 (4): 613–39.

Healey, B. J., and T. M. Evans. 2014. *Introduction to Health Care Services: Foundations and Challenges.* San Francisco: Jossey-Bass.

Healey, B. J., and M. Marchese. 2012. *Foundations of Health Care Management: Principles and Methods.* San Francisco: Jossey-Bass.

Johnson, C. E. 2009. *Meeting the Ethical Challenges of Leadership: Casting Light or Shadow,* 3rd ed. Thousand Oaks, CA: Sage.

Maurer, R. 1996. *Beyond the Wall of Resistance: Unconventional Strategies That Build Support for Change.* Austin, TX: Bard.

*Merriam-Webster Collegiate Dictionary.* 2016. "Trust." Accessed February 11. www.merriam-webster.com/dictionary/trust.

Morrison, E. E. 2011. *Ethics in Health Administration.* Boston: Jones & Bartlett.

Simons, T. 2002. "The High Cost of Lost Trust." *Harvard Business Review* 80 (9): 18–19.

# ORGANIZATIONAL CULTURE BUILDING

# THE PROCESS OF CULTURE DEVELOPMENT IN HEALTHCARE ORGANIZATIONS

Bernard J. Healey

## Learning Objectives

After completing this chapter, the reader should be able to

- discuss the importance of a strong, positive culture in healthcare organizations;
- explain the process of culture development in organizations;
- describe the steps required to perform a culture audit; and
- understand the leader's role in the development and maintenance of a strong, positive culture in a healthcare organization.

## Key Terms and Concepts

- Climate
- Culture audit
- Culture building
- Informal leader
- Internal culture
- Results pyramid
- Stewardship
- Subculture
- Thick positive culture

## Introduction

Before beginning a discussion of **culture building**, we should consider why culture is important for businesses, especially healthcare businesses. Successful companies in the United States are able to learn the value of culture building early in their development. They have discovered that the leader is successful in goal achievement, and the company is profitable if the employees are all working in a **climate** supportive of their organization and personal growth. These companies realize from their inception that neither management

**Culture building**
The leader's activities related to creating a strong working climate for employees.

**Climate**
The attitude that workers have regarding the work they do and the organization they perform that work for.

nor leadership is the answer to success on its own. They recognize that all employees must work together for both short-term and long-term success. The best-run companies in the United States discover early in their operations that having a strong culture allows them to consistently outperform their competitors over time.

These abilities also pertain to healthcare organizations, where solid teamwork is essential to successful patient outcomes.

High-performing healthcare organizations no longer operate in a bureaucratic organizational structure because they have decentralized. They no longer have a book of rules and regulations to guide individuals' daily performance. They have their cultural—better yet, a common-sense—road map of the way things are done at this organization. In this context is where the true value of a **thick positive culture** comes into play. Successful companies all have their particular internal understanding of how to deliver healthcare services to their respected customers. To keep growing the healthcare culture, the leader needs to keep communicating a compelling vision to employees every day.

**Thick positive culture**
A working climate that supports excellence and is widespread throughout the organization.

## Defining Organizational Culture

According to Nahavandi (2015), the organizational culture involves the numerous beliefs and values held by a group of individuals. It represents the collection of behaviors exhibited by members of an organization passed on to new members as they become a part of the organization. The culture of an organization is considered a permanent fixture because it does not change often or easily. In fact, if the previous leaders "got culture right" in the first place, successive leaders have no need to change it. The need does exist, however, to ensure that the culture remains in tune with the organization's purpose and values. This is one of the most important reasons for a new leader to complete an audit of the organizational culture before attempting to change that culture. (The culture audit is discussed in detail later in the chapter.)

Belasen, Eisenberg, and Huppertz (2016) argue that the types of culture found in most organizations are resistant to change. Scott and colleagues (2003) point out that paying attention to the development of a thick positive culture is critical for healthcare organizations attempting to deal with healthcare reform, considering culture change is usually required for reform to be successful. Furthermore, healthcare organization leaders must understand the relationship between the culture and the performance of the organization after the change is introduced. They also need to grasp early in their tenure that culture change and development are among the most important responsibilities and are indicators of a strong leader.

In their classic work, Kotter and Heskett (1992) suggest conceptualizing the organization as having two levels of culture: one completely visible and one less visible. The more visible culture highlights the behaviors that new employees are encouraged to follow. These values usually are not difficult to change. The less visible level of culture represents the shared values that typically are seen over the long term in an organization. These values are difficult to change because they are essentially hidden but at the same time are felt and shared by most members of the organization.

The hidden culture is where the **informal leader** plays a key role. The formal or titled leader needs to not only be aware of the informal leader's influence but also tap that individual's power to mobilize the underlying culture toward strong and positive change.

**Informal leader**
An individual who has developed power without being an appointed manager.

## How Culture Develops

Group culture develops over a long period through a trial-and-error process until the majority of group members feel comfortable with the culture.

When a business is first launched, the culture is given life by the founder and his first few hires. As the company grows and becomes profitable, new workers are hired and absorbed into the culture. The key at this stage, which many corporate leaders fail to realize, is to continue to pay a great deal of attention to the workers and their personal growth along with the development of the organization's culture.

An earlier take on culture development by Kotter and Heskett (1992) suggests that culture formation requires only that a group of people get together over time and be successful at what they do. If they solve problems during their time together, the solutions they used become a part of their specific culture. However, solutions that have been repeatedly successful tend to become deeply rooted in the culture and thus difficult to pull from it. This is the case in healthcare organizations. They have done things a certain way for a long period and been successful; they question why change is necessary even though their old solutions are no longer successful in dealing with today's problems.

Often, a poor culture can develop in reaction to negative views held by the employees concerning their personal growth and opportunities with the company. According to Lindgren (2012), designing a culture that supports the overall strategy of the organization is a proven key to successful outcomes. The vision articulated by the leader is aligned with the culture and the actions of the business. Employees are only willing to change past successful practices when they see a viable future in the new way of doing business.

The concept of subcultures in organizations is another facet of culture development. A **subculture** is a group of individuals in a culture that holds different beliefs from the overarching culture while maintaining some of its beliefs. Specifically, Schein (2004) has found that as organizations prosper and age, they form smaller units (subcultures) designed to cater to their distinct beliefs. These subcultures have their own leader, who articulates these beliefs. One type of subculture found in healthcare is based on occupation, such as physicians and nurses: Each group operates in the larger environment of a healthcare organization but develops specific, distinct roles—and beliefs attached to those roles—to be played in delivering healthcare services.

**Subculture**
A part of an organization that holds some beliefs that vary from those of the parent culture.

# Building Organizational Culture

Scott and colleagues (2003) have attributed an organization's failure to change its culture to inadequate or inappropriate leadership. They discovered that transactional and transformational leadership styles were most effective for driving cultural change, offering further support that culture shifts and development are related to leadership style. Therefore, the autocratic style of leadership in healthcare has given way to a more participative style to deal with a changing environment.

## Culture of Excellence

White and Griffith (2016, 19) argue that healthcare organizations need to concentrate on building a cultural foundation of excellence on five elements: "shared values, empowerment, communication, service excellence, and rewards for success." Combined, these elements represent the key for the leader to unlock the secret of building a culture than can embrace change and direct it toward organizational success. They also hold an attraction for employees who want to grow the organization as well as experience personal growth in their daily work.

### Shared Values

The first element of a culture of excellence relates to the shared values of all the stakeholders of the healthcare organization. As mentioned in an earlier chapter in terms of delivering the best healthcare possible to consumers, this element is important for the vast majority of individuals working in healthcare today. In other words, the shared values involved in helping others are among the most compelling reasons they dedicated their lives to delivering healthcare services to their patients.

## Empowerment

Many US healthcare organizations claim to practice empowerment, the second element of a culture of excellence. In actuality, their workers continue to function in an environment riddled with bureaucratic rules and regulations. True empowerment means the leader shares her power with the employees because the workers are closer to the customer than the leader is, and know better what those customers need on a daily basis. If an individual is empowered, he usually becomes motivated to deliver excellent care (recall the discussion on intrinsic motivation in chapter 4).

## Communication

The third element of a culture of excellence is the communication system established by the leader throughout the organization. Daily communication between leadership and staff makes a high-reliability organization special in that the communications move both ways. In fact, the leader of an organization with a culture of excellence spends more time listening to customers and staff than talking. In this way, the leader maintains constant awareness of those areas of concern customers and employees think are most important.

## Service Excellence

Service excellence emerges when an organization spends the majority of its time and energy offering service to customers that is not only exceptional but also attempts to be enhanced every day. The service excellence component of a culture of excellence can only be achieved through constant communication between customers and leaders and between leaders and staff. The key here is for the staff to be empowered to improve processes and execution without receiving approval from others in the organization. In other words, service excellence requires teamwork, constant communication, and worker empowerment all designed around daily improvement of service delivery.

## Rewards for Success

The last element of cultural excellence is concerned with the rewards for success in the way customers and staff are treated at the healthcare facility. According to White and Griffith (2016), a rewards-based culture of excellence represents the **stewardship** of the organization. The common belief found in a culture of excellence driven by rewards for success is that mutual support is fundamental to operations, such that teams support the overall organization and its leadership, and leaders support the teams in delivering excellent care and service to their customers. A culture of excellence characterized by mutual support grows stronger, thicker, and more positive every day.

**Stewardship**
The responsible management of scarce resources.

## Culture Change and Market Competitiveness

Connors and Smith (2011) suggest that most leaders are aware that moving the culture of their organization toward excellence can be instrumental in leading the competition. One important component of healthcare organizational culture change is the ability to markedly improve the organization's value proposition, thereby separating excellent organizations from good organizations. Correspondingly, an important task of leadership in culture shifts is to improve the value proposition offered by the healthcare system to the consumer of healthcare services. As mentioned earlier, this improvement requires the leader to facilitate service excellence by talking with and listening to employees and customers and empowering employees to do what is necessary to improve service delivery on a daily basis.

## The Role of Thick Culture in Building Organizational Culture

Southwest Airlines and SAS, discussed in an earlier chapter, are examples of strong, thick, positive cultures led by leaders who understand the importance of culture development and its relationship to organizational success.

A strong, thick, and positive culture features workers who thrive on intrinsic motivation that can often be sparked by a challenging work environment. Rework America (2015), in its book *America's Moment*, points out the danger inherent in subscribing to the so-called O-ring theory, named after the cause of the tragic loss of the space shuttle *Challenger* and all the souls aboard. The accident resulted from the failure of one small component, an O-ring, among thousands of parts in the space shuttle. The O-ring theory reveals an important lesson for industries such as healthcare: Organizations that produce complex products by their nature require that quality and skills intertwine in such a way that they cannot be understood through simple analysis. All it takes is one small mistake to ruin the entire production process. One example of this problem in healthcare is the fact that improper hand-washing techniques can cause a disease outbreak in a healthcare facility.

Such challenges can be addressed and overcome in a culture that supports key aspects of creativity and problem solving, which taps staffs' intrinsic motivation. Csikszentmihaly (2009), for example, points out that the development of flow in employees' work allows staff to feel a type of joy when their work is challenging. People appreciate work that is challenging and at the same time offers rewards they cannot get with free time. Individuals also like working with the team to meet these challenges. Therefore, the ideal culture may be a shared network designed by both leaders and followers to meet the challenges of work. Here, the culture not only helps ensure that the challenges are met but also produces intrinsic motivation for all the employees involved in the challenge.

The concept of flow at work has proved to be an important revelation for leaders in healthcare organizations because it reveals a way to engage the employee that is necessary to meet the challenges facing the healthcare industry. The leader should spend a great deal of time helping followers achieve their flow, which should ultimately improve healthcare delivery while creating intrinsic motivation for his followers. Part of that commitment involves understanding and appreciating the importance of flow and intrinsic motivation as part of the organization's **internal culture**. To achieve this understanding and appreciation, however, the leader first must understand the value of intrinsic motivation at work in healthcare and learn how to provide it for healthcare employees who are focused on navigating the potentially massive change to the way they do their work.

> **Internal culture**
> The values and beliefs of a business that are found deep within the organization.

## The Value of Culture in Healthcare

In recent years, we have heard and read much about the importance of culture to organizational growth and longevity. Culture and its value are sought-after topics at business conferences, and interest seems to be growing in organizational culture as a potential remedy for failing to keep up with the ongoing technological changes in society and industry.

This interest is expanding even though we know culture is an abstraction. Why do we have more interest in culture now than in years past, and what is the value of culture for organizational performance?

The answers to these questions is found in the rapidly changing business environment and the need for dedicated employees who constantly innovate the way products are made and services are delivered. These changes are forcing the vast majority of businesses and their employees to question everything they do to improve service delivery. This questioning process, along with a hardwired process for innovation, should be part of every organizational culture.

### *The Role of Inquiry in Adaptation*

Berger (2014) argues that many organizational cultures do not tolerate questioning because it distracts from productivity and because questioners tend to expect immediate answers, which leaders are either unable or unwilling to accommodate. In many bureaucratic organizations, lower-level employees are not allowed to ask questions of higher-authority-level individuals.

This type of policy is detrimental to growth and devalues the importance of culture. Especially in these times of change and uncertainty, healthcare organizations should be questioning everything they do and why. Those that block a culture founded on inquiry because they do not want to spend time defending proven methods forget that past success does not guarantee future success. The only way to adjust to changing market conditions and disruptive innovation is by instilling a questioning culture designed to foster creativity and adaptive flows.

As noted by Rework America (2015), those who work on the front lines in healthcare delivery are marginalized and even ignored in the inquiry process as organizations attempt to improve service delivery. As a counter-argument to this culture-driven marginalization, it provides an excellent example of the use of a culture of inquiry in *America's Moment*. The Para-professional Healthcare Institute (PHI) of New York provided training to frontline workers to improve the process of healthcare delivery in the home setting in response to staff feedback induced by an inquiry process. The orga-nization equipped home health workers with tablet computers for their visits to homes and trained the staff to assess client health risks and coordinate the sharing of results with the rest of the healthcare team. One adjustment made as a result of this initiative was for home health workers to administer client assessments consisting of 15 questions concerning their health at a given time. The findings from the questionnaires are then shared with other medi-cal professionals, helping to ensure continuity of care—a key component of value-based reimbursement. The result of the effort was a much lower use of the affiliated health system's emergency department than in the past, sav-ing money for the healthcare organization. This innovation, and the inquiry process that drove it, became part of the culture of PHI.

## Changing Culture in Healthcare

A number of avenues are available to leaders who recognize the need to promote a thick positive culture in their organization. In this section, we describe the culture audit, some building blocks for creating a thick culture, and the results pyramid. Later, we discuss the healthcare leader's role in cul-ture change.

### The Culture Audit

Before attempting any efforts at culture change, the leader of an organiza-tion must understand the culture currently in place. This effort can be an exhausting process and requires the leader to have the patience to gather data concerning the cultural manifestations present in the organization.

**Culture audit**
A formal investigation of the culture of an organization.

The leader may think she understands the current culture of the organization, but she needs to verify her assumptions before attempting the process of cultural change through a **culture audit**. The culture audit is a structured means to assess the sentiments of organizational members using a series of predetermined questions developed to reveal meaningful clues about the existing culture.

If the need for culture change is isolated, Schein (2009) recommends conducting a culture audit by seeking the input of members of the group that needs to change.

Although many outside experts are available to help complete a cultural audit, research conducted by Schein (2004) indicates that leaders should conduct their own audit of the current culture. They may begin by focusing on what behaviors surprised or stood out to the leaders when they first arrived at the organization.

The next step is to ask a recent hire to describe his impressions of working for the company. What surprised him as he began this new work? During this phase of the audit, leaders should focus on surprises for the new employee concerning the operations of the organization. They also may be able to discover which staff members tend to serve as the informal leaders. This time with the new hires and informal leaders is well spent, as the surprises and concerns they mention may well be the foundations of the organization's culture.

To gain further depth of insight from the culture audit, leaders also may identify particularly motivated individuals to determine their sources of motivation and the extent to which such motivation is normal for staff at the organization.

Having discussions with as many members of the facility as is feasible adds quality to the audit data, as does gaining access to the thoughts of informal leaders. For example, an informal leader may have an explanation for the surprises expressed by new hires. Leaders may wish to explore the organizational surprises with the informal leader and an organized focus group of staff to discover why they are considered surprises, why the events occur in the organization, or other key questions.

This questioning process typically leads to the development of a hypothesis as to why activities are conducted the way they are. This hypothesis then triggers an investigation to assess its truth.

Another area that should be covered in the culture audit is the presence of artifacts that characterize the organization (Schein 2009). New employees are more likely to discuss artifacts than behaviors or processes that surprised them. These could be items such as the communications process in the organization; the types and frequency of social events; the way conflicts are handled; the dress code; and the formality of relationships, especially between the leader and staff.

Finally, as they become increasingly experienced, leaders should periodically conduct benchmark comparisons against successful companies both inside and outside of healthcare to determine how their cultures match up.

For example, a large number of organizations that have been successful in recruiting talented individuals credit their success to tight screening processes. This type of employee screening includes multiple interviews with different individuals to determine if the potential employee fits the culture of the organization. Because questioning is considered an important success factor in today's turbulent environment, the candidate may be asked to bring questions to the interview.

Many successful companies over the years have embedded celebrations of success into their culture. Stories and myths develop around these celebrations that help the workers feel they are part of one big family at work. Most people enjoy celebrating positive outcomes and events, and the way these celebrations are conducted in the workplace becomes an important aspect of developing a strong positive culture. It shows workers that their performance as employees and team members is appreciated by the leader of the organization, and it offers motivation to continue performing at a high level.

### The Building Blocks of a Thick Healthcare Culture

Significant research shows that strong, thick, and positive cultures are directly related to both short- and long-term success. What are the required building blocks of a thick positive healthcare culture? Ledlow and Coppola (2011) make a convincing argument that thick positive cultures are often the result of employees learning how to solve problems as a team. Schein (2004) agrees that thick culture formation is usually the result of shared basic assumptions that have a history of past success in problem solving. Dolan (2010) believes that all the requisite skills for improved excellence in organizations cannot be found in one individual but are available in a team approach to solving problems.

Many who work in healthcare delivery dedicate their life to serving others. This position is an excellent starting point for not only a thick positive culture but also a performance-based culture because of the important work healthcare staff do every day. Members of a performance-based culture do not allow their customers to be hurt by the procedures that are meant to help them, and the healthcare leader supports their efforts by facilitating workers' return to a positive flow in their work processes when they are disrupted.

However, many individuals who have entered employment in healthcare have had their dreams of service and personal growth blocked time after time. Numerous healthcare organizations still rely on the bureaucratic organizational structure, filled with rules and regulations and micromanagement, which blocks innovation and employee empowerment.

Therefore, a second building block for a thick positive culture is the foundation of a decentralized organizational structure that relies on employee empowerment to make common-sense decisions. A structural shift of such magnitude requires that healthcare managers accept a certain amount of power loss, which can introduce resistance to change. Leaders must anticipate political or other types of resistance to rebuild the appropriate culture for meeting the future challenges in healthcare delivery.

A third powerful building block is the presence of a learning environment in which all staff are encouraged to educate themselves and grow to meet future demands. The strongest cultures normally have some supported educational initiatives designed to help their employees develop. Tuition reimbursement programs are not necessarily the best incentives for employees because many may already have advanced degrees and are not interested in adding more diplomas to their resume. They are, however, usually interested in training and development programs that will help them perform their job better.

A final building block of strong, thick, positive cultures is the provision of different types of buy-in mechanisms selected by employees. For example, many successful companies that have built strong, positive cultures offer stock purchase programs to their employees, in effect making them part owners of the company. Such gestures toward instituting the empowerment of employees only strengthens the culture.

## The Results Pyramid

According to Connors and Smith (2011), a simple method for changing the culture of the organization is the **results pyramid**. This model concentrates on the most important aspects of an organization's culture: experiences, beliefs, and actions. Specifically, "experiences foster beliefs, beliefs influence actions, and actions produce results" (Connors and Smith 2011, 22). The leader needs to understand the internal culture of his organization. The culture that has been developed in your organization is designed to produce your results. If the results are not acceptable, the culture needs to be changed to improve the results.

**Results pyramid**
A model of culture change that concentrates on the most important parts of the organization.

Furthermore, Schein (1988) points out that gaining an understanding of culture helps leaders recognize some of the irrational behaviors practiced by people in a given organization. One example of an irrational organizational behavior is when healthcare workers fight among themselves over necessary changes—the nature of the changes, how best to implement them, whether they are needed at all, and so on—when they should be collaborating on delivering enhanced services to their patients. Another type of irrational organizational behavior is seen when industries disrupted by much smaller organizations knew the change was coming and ignored it. In fact, many of these disrupted companies also had the answer that could have saved their business if they had only implemented it before the start-up company did. A good example of irrational behavior by members of an organization is seen in the decline of Eastman Kodak Company, which had initially developed the technology for an innovative type of film but failed to act on this success, thereby causing the company to go bankrupt.

## The Leader's Role in the Improvement of Culture

The healthcare leader must pay attention to building a strong organizational structure every day through her communication skills and by establishing trust. The majority of employees will support the leader in her efforts as long as they know what is being done and why. According to White and Griffith (2016), the highest-performing healthcare organizations implement the seven functions shown in exhibit 7.1.

Exhibit 7.1 explains the many functions of cultural leadership and demonstrates the alignment of the important functions with their intent and implementation. It also offers real-world examples of each function in the workplace. Interesting to note is that many of these functions are practiced at the same time by employees as by managers.

One step often overlooked by organizations eager to achieve high performance is that leaders should make certain the current culture cannot achieve the desired or required results (Connors and Smith 2011). In healthcare, the question is, "Can we reduce costs and improve the quality of services with the current culture?" If the answer is no, then and only then should the leader begin the long and difficult process of changing the culture of the organization.

Connors and Smith (2011) also point out that changing the culture of an organization cannot be turned over to other people or other departments; it is a function of the leader. Furthermore, the earlier the change process is begun, the healthier will be the culture that emerges. Cultural change is a continuous process of constant fine-tuning by the leader.

### The Importance of Staff Development in Culture Change Efforts

The most important component in the delivery of healthcare services is the people who deliver the services to their customers. If these individuals are satisfied with their work and provided the appropriate resources to complete it, they are capable of delivering extraordinary services.

Despite that truism, a shocking number of leaders in healthcare organizations fail to be concerned about the professional development of their employees. Empowering all employees is a first step in the development of the people working in a healthcare organization. Once empowered, staff also are capable of offering ideas for the improvement of many processes in the delivery of healthcare services because they provide these services daily. They now are part owners in the processes being improved, making the satisfaction of employees one of the most important aspects of a strong, positive culture. Motivated employees usually remain with a company longer and exhibit

| Function | Intent | Implementation | Examples |
|---|---|---|---|
| Promoting shared values | Establishes a central moral focus<br>Protects individual rights<br>Creates an intrinsic reward | Visioning exercises<br>Display and repetition<br>Training<br>Repetitive modeling<br>Rewards | Mission/vision/values on badges<br>Orientation emphasis<br>Celebration of exceptional effort |
| Empowering associates | Strengthens associate self-image<br>Encourages continuous improvement<br>Promotes responsiveness to customers | Training<br>Manager training<br>Repetitive modeling<br>Rewards | Demonstrated mastery of work procedures<br>360-degree manager assessments<br>Associate roles on PITs<br>Encouragement |
| Communicating with associates | Identifies and responds to concerns<br>Prevents information loss | Manager training<br>Meeting management<br>Display and repetition<br>Repetitive modeling<br>Rewards | Reports on goal achievement<br>Rounding<br>Blogs and e-mails<br>PITs and group meetings |
| Supporting service excellence | Focuses associates on meeting customer needs | Goal setting<br>Operational management<br>Training<br>Repetitive modeling<br>Rewards | Goal negotiations<br>Reports on goal achievement<br>Customer relations training<br>Service rewards and celebrations |
| Encouraging, rewarding, and celebrating success | Reinforces appropriate behavior<br>Builds associate loyalty | Performance measurement<br>Celebrations<br>Incentive compensation | Patient satisfaction<br>"Caught in the Act" program<br>Bonuses |
| Developing and sustaining the leadership team | Ensure that the organization has adequate leaders and "bench strength" | Routine leadership assessment, individual development plans, and a leadership succession plan | High potentials program; executive coaching; leadership academies |
| Improving the transformational culture | Increases return from culture over time | Review of learning, perceptions, attitudes, and achievements | Better programs to assist new leaders<br>Improvement of incentive system |

**EXHIBIT 7.1**
Functions of Cultural Leadership

*Source:* White and Griffith (2016). Reprinted with permission. PIT = performance improvement team.

better corporate citizenship behavior while working for the company than those who are unmotivated to perform.

This is a critical piece of knowledge for leaders to understand if they wish to build a culture that can successfully deal with all the changes to come in the delivery of healthcare services. Motivated employees and a strong positive culture go hand in hand, and keeping staff motivated helps an organization retain its talented employees so they do not take leave, perhaps taking their skills to a competitor.

Many proven methods are available to develop staff in healthcare organizations. The starting point is usually for the leader to show every day that he believes in the people who work for the organization. Businesses that have developed cultures focused on enhanced performance take pride in their workers and customers and seek to never bring harm to either group. This seems like such an easy path to follow, yet many organizations have yet to learn this lesson. Far too many leaders fail to understand how important staff development is to culture building. Successful companies all seem to have the same basic acknowledgment of the value of their people and their customers. They realize that if they work hard at developing their people by enabling them to improve their performance, everyone in the organization, including their customers, benefits.

## Implementing Cultural Change in Healthcare Organizations

Scott and colleagues (2003) have found that cultures that emphasize teamwork and coordination are associated with the continuous improvement of quality in care delivery. Cultures that are absorbed informally and that operate under bureaucratic rules and regulations perform poorly in quality improvement. The evidence from Scott and colleagues highlights one more reason healthcare services organizations must undergo severe shifts in culture. This mandate must be carried out by the leader who is capable of working with her staff to implement widespread cultural change in healthcare organizations as soon as possible.

The goals of leadership in healthcare organizations for the next several years will be to reduce the costs of care and improve the quality of services. These two important goals need to be embedded into the culture of healthcare organizations, and to do so requires evidence-based management (EBM).

To move toward accomplishing these goals, Joshi and colleagues (2014) recommend the use of the evidence-based leadership framework developed by the Studer Group and shown in exhibit 7.2.

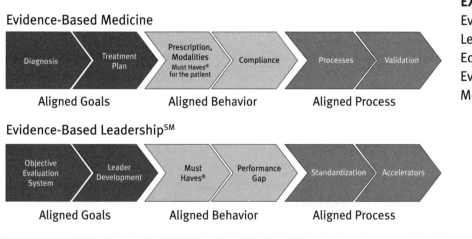

**EXHIBIT 7.2**
Evidence-Based
Leadership
Echoes
Evidence-Based
Medicine

*Source:* Studer Group LLC. Reprinted with permission.

Exhibit 7.2 shows how evidence-based leadership and evidence-based medicine are joined in one model to form EBM. The model also includes a comparison of each model in terms of aligned goals, aligned behavior, and aligned process. The EBM model is a framework for gathering as much evidence as possible concerning the risks and benefits of medical interventions to help in medical decision making. Although a simple process, EBM is a time-consuming model to institute. Once in place, however, it allows healthcare providers to make clinical decisions that improve health outcomes at a reasonable cost while not harming the patient.

EBM codifies the use of behaviors that have had the greatest success on patient outcomes, which should then be woven into the culture of the healthcare organization.

## Summary

To deal with the major problems facing healthcare delivery today, organizational leaders need to learn the value of culture building toward performance improvement. Neither management nor leadership is the answer to success on its own; all employees must work together to achieve service excellence in both the short term and the long term.

Employees are the most important component of a strong, positive culture in an organization. Leaders who attempt to build the type of culture that can successfully deal with all the change to come in the delivery of healthcare services must recognize that motivated employees and a strong, positive culture go hand in hand.

The goal of healthcare organizations is to deliver the best healthcare services possible to every consumer at an affordable price. Because healthcare leaders cannot be involved in every decision required of the business on a daily basis, employees must be empowered in the true sense of the word, such that the leader shares decision-making authority with her staff. Staff development also plays a key role in facilitating culture change toward performance improvement.

## Discussion Questions

1. Explain what culture is and why it should be important to a leader.
2. Name and explain the functions of cultural leadership.
3. What are the components of a cultural foundation of excellence? Describe each component.
4. What is the role of the leader of a healthcare organization in culture building?

## References

Belasen, A., B. Eisenberg, and J. W. Huppertz. 2016. *Mastering Leadership: A Vital Resource for Health Care Organizations.* Burlington, MA: Jones & Bartlett Learning.

Berger, W. 2014. *A More Beautiful Question.* New York: Bloomsbury.

Connors, R., and T. Smith. 2011. *Change the Culture: Change the Game.* New York: Penguin.

Csikszentmihaly, M. 2009. *Flow.* New York: Harper Collins.

Dolan T. C. 2010. "Leadership Skills for Healthcare Reform." *Healthcare Executive* 25 (5): 6.

Joshi, M. S., E. R. Ransom, D. B. Nash, and S. B. Ransom. 2014. *The Healthcare Quality Book: Vision, Strategy, and Tools.* Chicago: Health Administration Press.

Kotter, J., and J. L. Heskett. 1992. *Corporate Culture and Performance.* New York: Free Press.

Ledlow, G. R., and N. Coppola. 2011. *Leadership for Healthcare Professionals: Theory, Skills and Applications.* Burlington, MA: Jones & Bartlett.

Lindgren, M. 2012. *21st Century Management: Leadership and Innovation in the Thought Economy.* New York: Palgrave Macmillan.

Nahavandi, A. 2015. *The Art and Science of Leadership,* 7th ed. New York: Pearson.

Rework America. 2015. *America's Moment: Creating Opportunity in the Connected Age*. New York: W. W. Norton.

Schein, E. H. 2009. *The Corporate Culture Survival Guide*. San Francisco: Jossey-Bass.

———. 2004. *Organizational Culture and Leadership*, 3rd ed. San Francisco: Jossey-Bass.

———. 1988. *Organizational Culture and Leadership*. San Francisco: Jossey-Bass.

Scott, T., R. Mannion, H. T. O. Davies, and M. N. Marshall. 2003. "Implementing Culture Change in Health Care: Theory and Practice." *International Journal for Quality in Health Care* 15 (2): 111–18.

White, K. R., and J. R. Griffith. 2016. *The Well-Managed Healthcare Organization*, 8th ed. Chicago: Health Administration Press.

# THE PROCESS OF CHANGE IN HEALTHCARE ORGANIZATIONS

Bernard J. Healey

## Learning Objectives

After completing this chapter, the reader should be able to

- understand the major challenges of the changing healthcare environment,
- understand the need for change in the way the US healthcare system responds to the country's chronic disease epidemic,
- recognize the value of managing the change process, and
- understand the importance of involving all employees in the change process.

## Key Terms and Concepts

- Bundled payment system
- Capitation
- Change management
- Digital support system
- Health education programs

- Illness system
- Intermediary
- Passive resistance
- Patient-centered healthcare
- Sense of urgency

## Introduction

The beginning of the twenty-first century seemed to have set the stage for a sea change in every US industry. The changes have continued to multiply as technology expands the boundaries of the possible. In recent years, multiple factors have caused the largest industry in the United States, healthcare delivery, to face enormous change in a short period.

The biggest problem associated with a change in an organization is the tendency for its administrators not to involve everyone in the change process. Some upper-level leaders even strive to keep major changes secret, as parents would keep Christmas presents hidden from their young children. This approach makes no sense in any type of business because eventually, all stakeholders will know that change was discussed and even implemented without their input. Those who were not involved in the change process become resentful, leading to sometimes deep distrust in leadership. This distrust, in turn, causes a lack of interest in being part of the proposed or implemented changes.

**Passive resistance**
Noncompliance with authority; differentiated from active resistance by ignoring authority and not cooperating with requests for change.

If all staff do not support the change and **passively resist** the change process, the successful implementation of the change is virtually impossible.

Leaders in healthcare today, many of whom have come to recognize the importance of including staff in decision making surrounding change, are concerned about how to help their employees understand the need for change in the way they do business. Despite the inclination of employees and organizations to resist change, the relentless pace of change in the healthcare environment is only accelerating, and it will require organizations to hire and retain empowered and motivated employees capable of delivering superior services daily in a shifting context.

## Preparing for Change

**Sense of urgency**
A belief, evident in one's behavior, that action must be taken immediately.

Jennings (2012) indicates the need for leaders who both embody and create among others a **sense of urgency**. In times of change, that sensibility translates to the readiness, willingness, and ability to deal with the rapidly shifting environment that now defines healthcare delivery, especially in the face of disruptive innovation. The healthcare leader must constantly keep up with the evolutionary trends taking place and initiate her employees to the many examples of healthcare change found throughout the United States. By showing employees real-world examples of the changing healthcare environment, the leader helps prepare staff for the adjustments necessary for continued growth and, in some cases, survival.

Kotter (2012) argues that major change efforts are destined to produce some pain for all organizations and their staff; it cannot be avoided. The most common reason that change causes such a high degree of pain is that the organizations experiencing these difficulties were complacent in the implementation of change and never created a sense of urgency in members. The situation is no different with healthcare organizations, which must reduce costs, improve quality, and exploit environmental opportunities or fail in their mission. Before changes are implemented—and, ideally, before they are developed—the leader is responsible for making every staff member aware that change is coming and helping each understand the reasons specific changes need to be made sooner rather than later.

### Forget the Past

Lindgren (2012) suggests that forgetting the past and viewing the future as the starting point allows the healthcare leader to always be a few steps ahead of current and even future competitors. Among the steps he discusses in his process to shape the future is to perceive the future as offering numerous opportunities and continuous experiments. However, one cannot shape such a future if one does not know the forces of future change. Thus, we present a sampling of the many change forces now descending on the healthcare industry or anticipated in the future for the healthcare leader to consider.

### Be Selective in Areas of Early Focus

With so many change factors in the offing, deciding which to attend to becomes difficult. In the author's view, the forces shown in exhibit 8.1 are most likely to trigger major change for the healthcare industry in both the short term and the long term. These forces of change include the chronic disease epidemic, the role of third-party payers, the need for wellness programs, the onset of new financing mechanisms for healthcare, the new

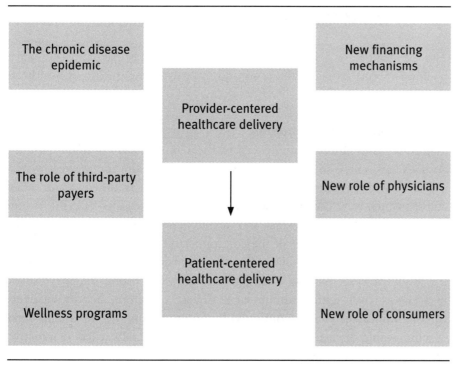

**EXHIBIT 8.1**
Forces of Future Change

role of physicians, the new role of consumers, and the call for a patient-centered healthcare system. Each of these areas is discussed in detail in the next section.

These forces of change have been ignored by many healthcare organizations in the past, but that stance is no longer feasible. In fact, some of these forces have already caused hospital closures or mergers throughout the United States. The healthcare industry has no choice but to deal with these forces of change successfully by designing or adopting a **change management** process (discussed in detail in a later section).

**Change management**
The thoughtful identification and implementation of new ways to accomplish goals.

Before we consider the impending forces of change in healthcare, a worthwhile question to pose is, Why were they ignored? Berger (2014) posits that so-called idle questioning is often seen by business executives as inefficient; they would rather take action, even if the wrong strategy is pursued. Each of the forces discussed is accompanied by an obvious proposed solution that has not been implemented. The lack of implementation signals the need for strong leadership and empowered followers to ask questions concerning an enhanced way to meet these challenges. Questioning of employees and customers must occur for healthcare leaders to discover potential solutions. At the same time, those being questioned should know that the plan is to evaluate all potential solutions with no guarantee that only the proposed answers will be considered.

## Factors in Determining the Need for Change

The US healthcare delivery system is in need of great change if the nation is serious about reducing the costs and improving the quality of healthcare for all.

### The Chronic Disease Epidemic

The patterns of disease experienced in the United States over the past few decades have changed dramatically. Early on, the healthcare delivery system was faced with communicable disease epidemics such as influenza and tuberculosis, which were capable of waging widespread disease and death. As time went on, healthcare providers and researchers developed treatments and control measures for many of the communicable diseases and improved the overall understanding of their modes of transmission. This movement toward the study of epidemiology and application of antiobiotic therapy resulted in a victory over acute communicable disease epidemics. As the incidence of communicable diseases continued to decrease, funding was pulled from communicable disease programs, resulting in future, albeit less destructive, outbreaks of communicable diseases.

The communicable disease epidemic was essentially replaced by an epidemic of chronic diseases that are capable of depleting all the money available to the healthcare sector at present. The chronic disease epidemic is unlike any other challenge faced by the US healthcare system simply because the system as a whole does not operate on an understanding of the long-term ramifications of this epidemic. Bland (2014) estimates that chronic diseases affect one out of two US residents and account for 80 percent of total healthcare costs annually.

Unlike communicable diseases, chronic diseases are not spread from person to person and, once acquired, are incurable. Chronic diseases also produce a great deal of suffering and disability, particularly due to the complications that may develop from having these diseases for a long period.

Stakeholders in the US healthcare system, from policy experts to observers to board members, leaders, clinicians, and staff, need to begin looking at the healthcare delivery system as a production process designed to keep people healthy. The current system is passive in that it requires individuals to seek care to maintain wellness or treat illness. The problem is that, by the time medical attention is sought, the chronic disease is likely established in the patient, prevention cannot take place, and no cure is available for the disease. The only course is tertiary prevention, which requires the patient to take action to prevent the long-term complications that usually result from chronic disease.

Instead, healthcare delivery as a production process can work to avoid this two-pronged prevention model. An example of how to be proactive with a chronic disease can be found in managing the epidemic of type II diabetes in the United States. This chronic disease can cause disability and lead to premature death if not handled effectively. Ideally, prevention efforts are undertaken to help individuals avoid acquiring this disease. One approach for individuals is to pretend that they have type II diabetes and do what is necessary to prevent onset and subsequent complications of the disease. Most of the activity involved in this approach does not even involve the healthcare system. The individual needs to maintain a healthy weight or lose weight by following an appropriate diet and getting lots of exercise. Visits to one's primary care physician complement these efforts to check on the patient's status. The point is that the same preventive behaviors as practiced to avoid complications, if practiced early and continuously, can prevent diabetes from ever occurring in the first place.

So if prevention of chronic diseases is so important, why do few healthcare systems spend their resources on **health education programs** designed to prevent chronic diseases from developing? Our current system of healthcare delivery is not designed to prevent anything. The system is designed to cure disease, a model that worked very well with communicable diseases. However,

**Health education programs**
Teaching strategies and tools designed to develop awareness in the population about good and bad health behaviors.

the healthcare system has never adapted to the occurrence of chronic diseases. Because the largest cost segment in the system consists of caring for chronic diseases, a tremendous need is evident for a new model to treat these diseases.

How the chronic disease epidemic is handled by the healthcare organization is one of the most important challenges facing the healthcare leader and his organization. The leader needs to be proactive in preparing his facility for the evolving nature of the chronic disease epidemic and its impact on the healthcare delivery system. One way to prepare is to participate in a series of discussions involving local public health departments concerning the extent of this epidemic and how healthcare facilities should address it.

### Third-Party Payers

**Intermediary**
An individual or organization that works between a buyer and a seller of a product or service.

Emanuel (2014) argues that health insurance companies—third-party payers—as we know them today are due for change. One of the architects of the Affordable Care Act, Emanuel believes that health insurance companies must change the way they do business or face extinction. Many health policymakers question the need for an **intermediary** between the consumer and the provider of healthcare, noting that the absence of a go-between would result in a less expensive way to pay for healthcare services. Third-party payers seem to have recognized the need for population-based prevention programs but devote few resources to ensuring a well-developed effort to prevent chronic diseases. For example, funds from insurers allocated to health education programs that begin in infancy and continue through individuals' working life would enhance population health, but they undercut insurers' own business over the long term.

However, to effect the type of change needed for the US healthcare delivery system, third-party payers must do much more than collect premiums and pay reimbursements. If they were to use their tremendous resources to help solve the chronic disease epidemic, they would add value to the healthcare system. Emanuel (2014, 319) predicts that "insurance companies will either become purveyors of management, analytics, and actuarial services or integrated delivery systems, actually employing (or contracting with) hospitals, physicians, and other providers to render patient care." This prediction, if realized, represents a major operational shift for every participant in the healthcare delivery system.

The demise of third-party payers may present a unique opportunity for many hospitals and health systems to exploit the changes and improve the system of care. Healthcare leaders must be proactive in anticipation of such disruption by holding regular discussions with staff regarding potential changes in reimbursement methods by third-party payers and how they can best prepare for the future of reimbursement for services.

## Wellness Programs

The ultimate goals of any healthcare consumer are usually to remain well and free of pain and disability and to lead a long life free of disease. Achieving the ideal healthcare system would help the consumer in this effort. However, the US medical care system operates as more of an **illness system**, as it typically delivers care only after consumers become ill and request treatment.

Now more than ever, consumers must take the initiative to remain healthy. As reimbursement incentives change, healthcare providers will be increasingly interested in offering wellness care to keep patients healthy because they will be paid for health outcomes rather than health activities, as was the case in the fee-for-service (FFS) scheme of reimbursement. With FFS, every time a physician completed a service or portion of a service, he was paid a certain amount for that service.

The area of wellness offers a prime opportunity to develop programs for preventing the occurrence of chronic diseases and complications from those diseases. The critical feature of a wellness program is that the patient take the lead role in maintaining wellness. A great deal of wellness activity is centered on avoiding high-risk health behaviors such as tobacco use, alcohol abuse, weight gain, and physical inactivity. This wellness regimen needs to be developed between the patient and her primary care physician.

Exhibit 8.2 shows how influential a healthcare organization can be in managing the health of the population. This model can be expanded to promote healthy behaviors for the entire population. It demonstrates the role healthcare organizations need to play in achieving and maintaining a healthy population, and it offers another good example of why hospitals and health systems need to acknowledge the fact that costs usually rise and individuals' stock of health decreases as they move away from a healthy state. The ideal preventive healthcare system will only become reality through strong leadership, and it must be in place as soon as possible. Resistance by those who profit from people becoming ill will not diminish until the US healthcare system has hardwired changes in which providers are paid entirely for outcomes rather than for activities. Wellness programs will support and promote these changes.

No quick fixes are available to eliminate or even reduce the high-risk health behaviors that have become part of our culture. Nonetheless, every effort should be made to educate the population about the dangers of chronic diseases and their complications over time. Escalating healthcare costs and poor quality of health are direct results of the explosion of chronic diseases in the US population; the prevention of high-risk health behaviors as a national policy must trump a medical model attempting to cure the incurable chronic diseases.

**Illness system**
An approach to care delivery that focuses on illness rather than wellness.

**EXHIBIT 8.2**
Personal
Services for
Community
Health

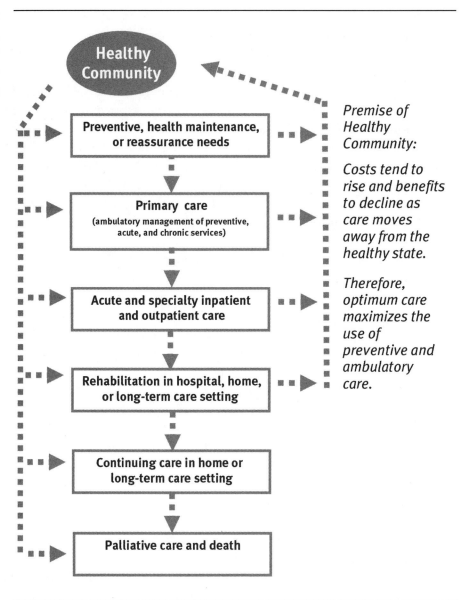

*Source:* White and Griffith (2016).

## *New Methods of Healthcare Financing*

Only people who support the current method of financing healthcare seem to benefit from this method. This is one area where almost everyone involved in healthcare research agrees that some type of change will occur shortly. Exhibit 8.3 demonstrates the explosion in federal healthcare spending as a proportion of total federal spending. This spending jumped from 12 percent in 1985 to 20 percent in 1995 and is projected to rise to 30 percent by 2018. When considered in the context of the large number of baby boomers

| | 1965 | 1975 | 1985 | 1995 | 2005 | 2012 | 2018* |
|---|---|---|---|---|---|---|---|
| Total federal spending | 118.2 | 332.3 | 946.3 | 1,515.7 | 2,472.0 | 3,537.1 | 4,449.2 |
| Federal health spending | 3.1 | 29.5 | 117.1 | 307.1 | 614.0 | 922.6 | 1,328.4 |
| Medicare | n/a | 12.9 | 65.8 | 159.9 | 298.7 | 471.8 | 614.8 |
| Medicaid | 0.3 | 6.8 | 22.7 | 89.1 | 181.7 | 250.5 | 390.6 |
| Veterans Administration | 1.3 | 3.7 | 9.5 | 16.4 | 28.8 | 50.6 | 60.3 |
| Other | 1.5 | 6.1 | 19.1 | 41.7 | 105.0 | 149.7 | 262.8 |
| Federal health spending as a percentage of total federal spending | 2.6% | 8.9% | 12.4% | 20.3% | 24.8% | 26.1% | 29.9% |

**EXHIBIT 8.3**
Federal Spending on Health, Fiscal Years 1965–2018 (in billions of dollars)

* Projected data; n/a: not applicable
*Source:* Reprinted from Feldstein (2015).

moving into Medicare and the increase in membership in the Medicaid program in recent years, the federal expenditures on healthcare over the next few years is clearly unsustainable. All stakeholders in the US healthcare system need to understand that the federal and state money being wasted on needless medical tests and medical procedures represents major opportunity costs, taking away funding for education, national defense, infrastructure, and a host of other very deserving federal and state government programs.

According to Feldstein (2015), the United States needs to become more avid in its efforts to reduce inefficiency in the provision and use of medical services. A high-efficiency system is becoming a priority for both the federal and state governments as the costs for healthcare continue to rise with no increase in the quality of healthcare being delivered.

An ideal way to finance healthcare delivery is through payment that encourages improved patient outcomes. Many proposals have been generated by health policy experts to enhance the population's health, including pay for performance, **capitation**, a **bundled payment system**, and payment for outcomes. If the healthcare financing system moves into a payment mechanism that encourages good health, there will certainly be a movement to improve the quality of services delivered to consumers. Incentives will also be in place to keep people healthy and free from chronic diseases through prevention programs.

### The New Role of Physicians

The role of the physician in the delivery of healthcare services is changing in many ways as the practice of medicine heads into an uncertain future. The

**Capitation**
A payment scheme by which a provider of healthcare is paid a set amount to deliver care for a certain period.

**Bundled payment system**
A reimbursement structure by which a single payment is made to two or more physicians for a particular episode of care.

physician's primary method of billing for services, FFS, gave him control over his income stream. In effect, the physician could create his own demand and then send in a bill and get paid for services rendered. This scheme evolved from the illness system mentioned earlier and allowed the physician to order and bill for medical services that had little or no value for the consumer's good health, and at times were dangerous, in addition to those that led to healing.

Thus, the need has never been greater for the development and acceptance of proven evidence-based healthcare services. And this aim is what comparative effectiveness research (CER) is designed to accomplish.

### Comparative Effectiveness Research

CER is a methodology used to determine the relative effectiveness, benefits, and potential harms of different treatment options. It applies rigorous analysis of the treatments' purported value compared to their costs. Because the healthcare delivery system has historically adopted expensive new products and services rapidly without conducting a thorough analysis of their value, this type of economic analysis helps leaders inform many of the decisions that now need to be made in this era of limited resources. For the leader of a healthcare facility attempting to reduce costs, this tool can be useful in eliminating waste and lowering costs of care. Despite the fact that providers may experience reduced reimbursements by limiting their services to those proven effective through CER, patients ultimately benefit, and the resulting improvements in patient population health should bring returns to the organization in the long term.

### Medical Education

Emanuel (2014) argues for a complete overhaul of medical school education to prepare physicians to deal with the new skills required for a successful practice in the future. Physicians must gain or enhance management skills, leadership skills, and communication skills. Probably the greatest deficit in physician training is in their knowledge of computers and information technology systems. In particular, Emanuel (2014) notes physicians will need comprehensive training or retraining in the use of electronic health records (EHRs) and in all types of **digital support systems**.

**Digital support system**
Suite of applications that work in conjunction with electronic health records.

## *The New Role of Consumers*

Futurists in healthcare delivery tend to ignore the role of the consumer when predicting the challenges to be faced by hospitals and health systems. But patients as consumers represent an emerging issue for organizations in a value-based reimbursement environment because they have historically been passive recipients of care in encounters with physicians and hospitals.

Patients have evolved into consumers in part because they are paying an ever-growing portion of the bill for healthcare services out-of-pocket. With increased cost has come increased scrutiny of the care consumers receive, and many patients have expressed dissatisfaction, concern, or unhappiness about the level of service they receive.

In addition, a great deal of medical information is now available for the consumer, thanks to the increased number and reach of news media outlets, the explosion of websites on disease-specific topics, and any number of friends and family eager to share their own newfound knowledge.

Topol (2015) envisions the physician–consumer relationship of the future as having the physician play the role of guide and navigator for the healthcare system, helping patient-consumers make the best decisions about their consumption of medical care services. With that shift, he sees the end of the doctor-dependent patient, replaced in many cases by the doctorless patient in the purchase and use of many medical services.

Topol's (2015) argument that patients have a greater part to play in their medical care than in the past is rooted in his belief that they are extremely smart about their body, and no one has a greater interest in their good health than they have. However, in part because of their training, many physicians still practice with an attitude of paternalism and may be dismissive of this type of smart patient. That attitude is destined to change as the smart patient becomes even smarter and more sophisticated in distilling that information.

## *Patient-Centered Healthcare Delivery*

Although the vast majority of Americans likely have never realized it, as patients they actually pay most of the cost of healthcare services, through their workplace, taxes, and out-of-pocket payments. They also take all the risks when they accept the care and treatment ordered by their physician.

Healthcare delivery in the United States was never designed to be a **patient-centered healthcare** system. According to Field (2014), the US healthcare system was created as a direct result of a collaboration between public (government) and private (hospitals and the American Medical Association) initiatives. Its core elements were shaped and developed by the federal government to be operated by private institutions. The average patient-consumer has not been included in the design and operation of the healthcare system she has long contributed to financially. This situation is changing, however, because the consumer of healthcare services is demanding representation in her healthcare decisions.

This new consumer leverage may represent the most important paradigm shift in the redesigned healthcare system. If the system becomes truly patient centered to include healthcare consumers' desires in the

**Patient-centered healthcare**
The provision of health services in a manner that is respectful of the patient's desires and expectations as well as clinical needs.

change process, a much improved system will be the result. However, most patient-consumers are not yet prepared to handle this responsibility. They must be educated to understand that their good health outcomes depend on their ability to make the right choices at the right times. They need to recognize, for example, that once they develop a chronic disease, fixing the problem—curing the disease—is not an option. Fortunately, healthcare leaders, care providers, and constituents can still manage this problem by working collaboratively.

## Change Management

The change process and change itself do not have to be the nightmare they are perceived to be for healthcare organizations. In fact, once undertaken, they should result in an improved system of medical care. The problem, of course, is not the long term but the short term, when all the pain of change is experienced. The overhaul of healthcare delivery requires leaders with a vision of what improvement looks like when the correct choices are made now.

### The Three-Stage Change Management Model

Lussier and Achua (2016) posit that one of the most popular models of change management is the force field model, developed by Kurt Lewin. It consists of three primary steps:

1. Unfreezing the current state
2. Completing a transformation to or moving toward a new state
3. Refreezing the new state

Each stage is discussed in detail in the following paragraphs.

Important to note here is that buried beneath this simplistic model are a number of components that fall under the leader's purview of responsibility. They include the learning process, the motivation process, and the process of collaboration. Considering the difficulties that change can usher in, the change process requires a great deal of planning. One frustrating aspect of today's turbulent healthcare environment is the continuous need for transformation: As rapidly as the organization changes, an almost immediate need presents itself to change again.

The unfreezing stage entails preparing for the change to be implemented and usually begins when the leader is convinced that the timing is appropriate to effect the optimal outcome. Nahavandi (2015) found that unfreezing the current state of the organization to allow change is the most difficult part of the change process. In this stage, the leader must recognize that, although some forces are likely to support the transformation, many more are in place to resist it. Leaders typically encounter difficulty influencing the unfreezing process because the managers who report to them tend to be more concerned with the present than they are with long-term plans. The leader must overcome this challenge by not only encouraging employees to think differently about the future but also nudging them toward helping the organization shift the way it conducts business to ensure future viability.

The second stage of change, the movement toward transformation, represents the actual shift to the types of change in behaviors and actions that need to be implemented in the organization. Nahavandi (2015) points to several areas of major change in business models that have been successful in the past but now must be adjusted to accommodate new technology, management practices, or other factors, requiring new skills for most employees as they respond to a highly informed consumer.

One example of the second stage of the change process is the adoption of EHRs. The EHR is an electronic replacement of the old paper record that contains patient health, treatment, and care information. This tool represents a significant shift in care delivery and health awareness for both the provider and the consumer. Hospitals, health systems, and physician offices benefit from the use of this virtual medical file or chart, which can be made available to all providers involved in a patient's care, ideally leading to reduction of medical errors and duplication of services. The patient-consumer benefits from electronic records because her medical information is now under her control, at least to some extent. EHRs are still considered a work in progress, but as with any change that is long overdue, perseverance is required to complete the transformation successfully and to the satisfaction of all stakeholders.

The transformational leadership style seems to work best in this second stage and is particularly critical to achieving success in effecting the needed transformation.

The final stage of the change process, refreezing, involves hardwiring the change into the operational system. To successfully refreeze the process, the leader must rely on his communication skills to help the organization's employees both accept and adapt to all of the changes. Staff are most likely changing years of habits that had probably worked well in the past. The leader must help employees embrace new behaviors and practices related to the change as the new way of conducting business.

Furthermore, the leader is instrumental in helping all his staff cement the newly changed behaviors in their individual business model. Ways that he can assist in this effort include providing applicable and adequate training; resources; and, in most cases, incentives for employees to fully adopt the new behaviors.

## The Nature of Change Management

Organizational change is never easy. It is made even more difficult for organizations that must operate under the types of rules and regulations required in the delivery of services, typically in the bureaucratic organizational structure. In the past, the change process was viewed as an enemy of the bureaucratic organization because managers often feared the loss of power. As leadership slowly replaces management in new organizational structures that are decentralizing control, the attitude toward change will move to acceptance and, eventually, anticipation and exploitation of change for organizational gain. Healthcare organizations must not only accept change but become proactive participants in the change process, initiating transformation to get ahead of cost escalation and quality improvement innovations.

Fried and Fottler (2015) characterize change management as being concerned with developing a response by the entire organization to external forces that threaten its survival. Exhibit 8.4 depicts a series of models that represent the components found in some of the best change models currently available.

This guide follows a seven-step process that begins with developing a compelling case for the change and ends with absorbing the change in the organization's culture. It offers numerous steps designed to engage the involvement of staff and help the leader manage potential resistance to the change, including a step for communicating with followers and one that calls for celebration upon the successful completion of the change process.

The beauty of the guide shown in exhibit 8.4 is that it takes into consideration some important components of the change process that are often overlooked in other models for managing change. For example, exhibit 8.4 notes the importance of sponsorship for the change by the C-suite and displays a step depicting integration of the changes into the culture of the organization.

## Launching the Change Process

To embark on a successful process of organizational change, the leader must grasp the significant implications of transformation in a bureaucratic organization. Many hospitals and health systems spend a great deal of time worrying about the change rather than working with staff to develop a response to the change. Too many facilities remain convinced that the winds of change are temporary and that, if they wait long enough, the need for transformation will diminish.

The healthcare leader must facilitate the change process while involving his followers to participate in it from the beginning and throughout each stage.

### Planning for Change in Healthcare Delivery

The successful healthcare leader develops a comprehensive plan for transformation before embarking on the process of change. An important starting

| Change Management Step | Description |
|---|---|
| 1. Compelling case and awareness | Make a compelling case for change to build awareness. Explain "why" before "how." Match communication style to audience preference. |
| 2. Sponsorship | Establish sponsorship for the change with an active leadership core to guide the effort. |
| 3. Involvement | Build involvement throughout. Identify key stakeholders and reach out to them. |
| 4. Project management | Create a plan and project management system to keep on track. |
| 5. Resistance management | Anticipate pushback and emotional reactions to change. Be sensitive to feelings of loss. Allow stakeholders to express emotional concerns. |
| 6. Communication and celebration | Communicate and celebrate results along the way. Don't wait for the complete change to take place. Celebrate quick wins. |
| 7. Cultural integration | Integrate changes into organizational culture. Hardwire the new way of doing things into key work processes and reward mechanisms. |

**EXHIBIT 8.4**
Leadership Guidance to Change Management

*Source:* Fried and Fottler (2015).

point that is often ignored is identifying the informal leaders in the organization. Informal leaders have power in the organization despite their lack of titled or positional influence. These individuals are usually respected by their fellow workers because of their personal power. When acknowledged and engaged, informal leaders can be a great help to the organizational leader in the change process.

A second step in planning for change is to ask staff a lot of questions and allow the employees as much time as they require to answer. This step represents an important part of the planning process in that it allows a period of digestion for all stakeholders to understand the urgency of change and offer their own ideas of what needs to be done, by whom, and when.

Another early step in the planning process should be to identify the training needs to ensure that the chosen type of change can be properly implemented in a timely fashion.

The transformation planning process in healthcare must be dynamic in that it continuously seeks to recognize the signs and symptoms of a changing environment. This process requires the leader to spend time discussing with all involved how to improve the patient experience in terms of hosting a guest at the healthcare facility. These continuous conversations with employees and customers should involve the leader knowing the right questions to ask and should be marked by more listening and less talking by the leader in these dialogues.

### Continuous Scanning of the Healthcare Environment

Healthcare facilities need to continually scan the entire healthcare environment, looking for opportunities that can be transformed into new methods for improving the services offered to consumers. The identification of opportunities can only be achieved by talking to employees and current customers to discover what services, types of encounters, responses, and other aspects of care they require. Organizational leaders are expected to maintain a keen awareness of the industry; healthcare staff should be empowered to undertake this effort as well.

Environmental scans are helpful in determining potential threats and opportunities that require appropriate responses by the hospital or health system. They build a forum in which to learn about changes in technology, reimbursement, competitors, and best practices in the delivery of healthcare services.

The attitude of anticipation for change has been among the weakest aspects of management in healthcare delivery because, as mentioned earlier, the manager traditionally is concerned with the current situation only. In a stable environment characterized by little environmental change, the manager attended to increasing efficiency and virtually ignored future threats to the organization. The so-called new normal, however, features a turbulent environment in which no leader has the luxury of complacency about future threats.

Another key aspect of environmental scans is their utility in identifying opportunities that can be exploited. For example, has the scan identified a particular service that is desired by a number of consumers that could be provided by the healthcare organization? Does a better approach exist for delivering a current service that would meet the needs of current customers more completely than the present method?

Belasen, Eisenberg, and Huppertz (2016) found that healthcare organizations are moving from a state of predictability to one allowing incremental change in response to an industry that now prominently features unpredictability. The new healthcare delivery system requires leaders who are future oriented and driven by industry observations (such as through environmental scanning) and capable of handling unpredictable external forces.

### Using Strategic Management

As discussed by Wheelen and colleagues (2015), the application of strategic management to organizational operations relies on decisions made by managers on how to best improve the long-term performance of a given organization. Strategic planning is concerned with financial planning, forecast-based planning, external planning, and strategic management. The sustainability of healthcare organizations in the future requires strategic management and planning processes, such as those mentioned earlier, to be implemented immediately to deal with the turbulent environment. Part of that strategic management approach for hospitals and health systems is to become learning organizations so that they are prepared for the change and can move forward proactively rather than reacting to developments. To do so, organizations must eliminate many of the features of a bureaucratic structure and thereby increase flexibility in their thinking and learning.

A prime example of the need for flexibility and agility in thinking is related to reimbursement. Altman and Mechanic (2015) point out that Medicare and Medicaid enrollments will have grown by 57 percent and 71 percent, respectively, from 2006 to 2022. At the same time, private-sector (nongovernmental) payers are experiencing approximately a 5 percent decline in enrollments. Private-sector insurers usually raise rates to compensate for decreased payments from the government. This relationship is shown in exhibit 8.5, whereby the government pays less than the cost of care in reimbursement, which is subsidized by private insurers paying more than the cost to make up for the government shortfall. However, this model of payment is no longer sustainable for numerous reasons, which include more people enrolling in government programs than in the past; less government money being available for reimbursement than under FFS; and the increasing inability of private payers to pay their costs, let alone subsidize Medicare and Medicaid payments. This trend will place tremendous pressure on healthcare facilities to reduce costs into the foreseeable future.

To reduce the costs of care delivery, organizations should apply their new understanding of what it means to be a learning organization and prepare for a transformed future, for example by moving from one strategy to another as the environment changes (Wheelen et al. 2015). Along the way, the learning organization creates new knowledge that it is equipped to readily share throughout the system. This knowledge helps the business remain creative, continue to innovate, and rigorously scan the environment for indications of additional change. This learning strategy is followed by leaders and followers using a feedback loop designed to keep everyone involved up-to-date on the situation.

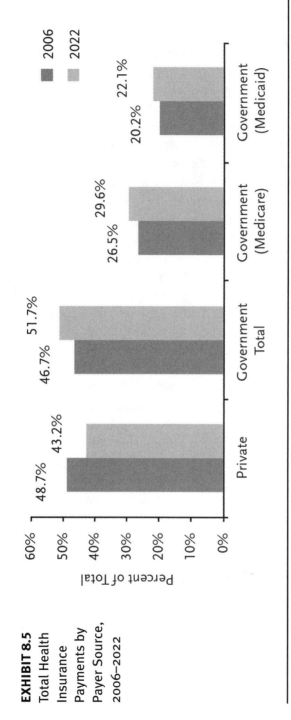

**EXHIBIT 8.5**
Total Health
Insurance
Payments by
Payer Source,
2006–2022

*Source:* Altman and Mechanic (2015).

# The Leader's Role in the Change Process

Kotter (2012) points out that when the leader is in the process of effecting change, she needs to create a powerful guiding coalition that develops a commitment to improved performance. This coalition is necessary to deal with the inevitable passive resistance that almost always happens when major change is being implemented.

## *Leadership Skills Required in the Process of Change*

Many leadership skills are necessary to guide the current healthcare delivery system through the changes necessary for survival in the turbulent healthcare environment.

### Communication of Transparency

Fifer (2015) asserts that many consumers of healthcare services are becoming frustrated that they cannot acquire reliable information about the cost of these services. Because people are now expected to pay more out-of-pocket for healthcare services than in the FFS era, they are demanding transparency in both price and quality. This expectation is forcing many healthcare systems to develop computerized transparency tools.

### Performance Improvement

According to Lawrence (2014), leaders of healthcare organizations need to determine how to achieve performance improvement while implementing innovations throughout their facility. Lawrence maintains that part of this effort includes conducting periodic assessments of how much progress is being made, with a consistent effort to improve healthcare delivery for all patients every day. The leader must drive home the point to every employee that the organization needs to attempt new activities and processes and take appropriate risks to make the improvement process work.

### Communication of Information to Staff

Unimpeded information flow in the organization is considered a prerequisite for successful transformation, but it also can produce negative consequences, such as jealousy among employees or customers comparing their level of service with other customers. The negative consequences can be reduced if the leader makes certain that the organization is transparent to all stakeholders of the business. With this understanding, the leader needs to spend much of his time sharing information with the employees about proposed changes and seeking their opinions about the ramifications of those changes.

### Setting of Priorities

Fullan (2011) indicates that when attempting to make change in any organization, the leader needs to focus on a small number of core priorities for achievement in the short term and then help the followers make the changes. Change is a collective process, with all players assuming equal importance in that process. Leading through transformation takes time and produces some pain, but it is worth the effort in the end.

## The Vagaries of Change Acceptance

Joshi and colleagues (2014) suggest that the science of innovation diffusion can offer an explanation as to why some innovations that cause change are immediately accepted while other innovative ideas are ignored. They indicate that rapid acceptance of innovations causing change depends on the relative advantage, compatibility, complexity, trialability, and observability of the change:

- The *relative advantage* is the belief that the new product or service is better than what it replaced.
- *Compatibility* is reflected in how the potential adopters react to the new item compared with what it replaces.
- The *complexity factor* is the perceived difficulty of using the innovation.
- *Trialability* is evident in the availability of the product or service on a trial basis before it must be adopted.
- *Observability* indicates the ability to view others attempting the change before they attempt it themselves.

## Summary

An important part of leadership in healthcare today is helping employees understand the need for change in the way they do business. Employees in healthcare tend to fear change and may not understand why their organizations need to transform, but despite their resistance, the pace of change in the healthcare environment is accelerating rapidly, making the adoption of change processes an imperative.

The process of change is never easy, and it is particularly difficult for organizations that deliver services. With bureaucracies now moving toward decentralizing control, the attitude toward change is shifting to acceptance and even exploitation. Healthcare organizations also need to continually scan the entire environment to determine new methods for improving the services offered to their consumers.

The process of change is a direct responsibility of both the leader and the followers of healthcare systems. Numerous ways are available to meet this responsibility, but most observers suggest leaders use the technique of questioning to discover the best solution.

## Discussion Questions

1. Name and explain some of the major challenges forcing healthcare organizations to realize the importance of transformation.
2. Offer a complete explanation of the process of change in organizations.
3. Explain how the leader in a healthcare organization should go about managing the process of change in his organization.
4. How can leadership help staff meet the challenges facing the redesigned healthcare delivery system in the United States?

## References

Altman, S. H., and R. E. Mechanic. 2015. "Limited Future Healthcare Spending Growth Will Force Providers to Develop More Cost-Effective Delivery Systems." In *Futurescan 2015: Healthcare Trends and Implications 2015–2020*, 4–9. Chicago: Health Administration Press and Society for Healthcare Strategy & Market Development.

Belasen, A., B. Eisenberg, and J. W. Huppertz. 2016. *Mastering Leadership: A Vital Resource for Health Care Organizations*. Burlington, MA: Jones & Bartlett Learning.

Berger, W. 2014. *A More Beautiful Question*. New York: Bloomsbury.

Bland, J. S. 2014. *The Disease Delusion: Conquering the Causes of Chronic Illnesses for a Healthier, Longer, and Happier Life*. New York: Harper Collins.

Emanuel, E. J. 2014. *Reinventing American Health Care: How the Affordable Care Act Will Improve Our Terribly Complex, Blatantly Unjust, Outrageously Expensive, Grossly Inefficient, Error Prone System*. New York: Public Affairs.

Feldstein, P. J. 2015. *Health Policy Issues: An Economic Perspective*, 6th ed. Chicago: Health Administration Press.

Field, R. I. 2014. *Mother of Invention: How the Government Created "Free Market" Healthcare*. New York: Oxford University Press.

Fifer, J. J. 2015. "Transparency: Meeting Expectations, Seizing Opportunities." In *Futurescan: Healthcare Trends and Implications 2015–2020*. Chicago: Health Administration Press and Society for Healthcare Strategy & Market Development.

Fried, B. J., and M. D. Fottler. 2015. *Human Resources in Healthcare: Managing for Success*. Chicago: Health Administration Press.

Fullan, M. 2011. *Change Leader: Learning to Do What Matters Most*. San Francisco: Jossey-Bass.

Health Administration Press (HAP) and Society for Healthcare Strategy & Market Development (SHSMD). 2015. *Futurescan: Healthcare Trends and Implications 2015–2020*. Chicago: HAP and SHSMD.

Jennings, J. 2012. *The Reinventors: How Extraordinary Companies Pursue Radical Continuous Change*. New York: Penguin.

Joshi, M. S., E. R. Ransom, D. B. Nash, and S. B. Ransom. 2014. *The Healthcare Quality Book: Vision, Strategy, and Tools*. Chicago: Health Administration Press.

Kotter, J. P. 2012. *Leading Change*. Boston: Harvard Business Review Press.

Lawrence, D. M. 2014. *Best Care, Best Future: A Guide for Healthcare Leaders*. Bozeman, MT: Second River Healthcare Press.

Lindgren, M. 2012. *21st Century Management: Leadership and Innovation in the Thought Economy*. New York: Palgrave Macmillan.

Lussier, R. N., and C. F. Achua. 2016. *Leadership: Theory, Application and Skill Development*, 6th ed. Boston: Cengage Learning.

Nahavandi, A. 2015. *The Art and Science of Leadership*, 7th ed. New York: Pearson.

Topol, E. 2015. *The Patient Will See You Now: The Future of Medicine Is in Your Hands*. New York: Basic.

Wheelen, T., J. D. Hunger, A. N. Hoffman, and C. E. Bamford. 2015. *Concepts in Strategic Management and Business Policy: Globalization, Innovation and Sustainability*, 14th edition. New York: Pearson.

White, K. R., and J. R. Griffith. 2016. *The Well-Managed Healthcare Organization*, 8th ed. Chicago: Health Administration Press.

# LEADING PEOPLE
# IN HEALTHCARE DELIVERY

# CONFLICT MANAGEMENT IN HEALTHCARE ORGANIZATIONS

Tina Marie Evans

## Learning Objectives

After completing this chapter, the reader should be able to

- explain the significance of workplace conflict,
- identify the most common causes of workplace conflict,
- discuss some of the costs of workplace conflict for the healthcare organization,
- examine the role of perception in interpersonal conflict,
- describe the most common conflict management styles,
- identify his or her personal conflict management style,
- distinguish among the seven strategies for conflict resolution, and
- articulate specific ways workplace conflict can be prevented.

## Key Terms and Concepts

- Cognitive response
- Conflict
- Conflict management style
- Interpersonal
- Interpersonal conflict
- Perception
- Physiological response
- Primary conflict tension
- Productivity

## Introduction

As a manager, one of your main responsibilities is to ensure that the members of your department work well together with a strong, collaborative team focus. With good leadership, workers accomplish the goals of the department and relate well on an **interpersonal** basis. Inevitably, however, even in

**Interpersonal skills**
Qualities that involve getting along with people.

**Conflict**
A serious and upsetting disagreement or argument between two or more individuals, typically over clashes in opinion, values, or actions.

situations when workplace operations are smooth and under control, conflict arises. A **conflict** is more than a simple disagreement; it is a situation in which employees perceive a threat—be it physical or emotional, whether to their sense of power or status—to their overall well-being.

Managers who regularly monitor the work environment notice conflicts quickly. Before responding to the situation, a good manager pauses to consider what caused the conflict; whether it could have been prevented; and, now that it has arisen, how to address it in a timely way to limit any damage the conflict may cause. A study by Lang (2009) found that managers spend more than 18 percent of their time handling employee conflicts in the workplace, making conflict a significant managerial concern with a high time and productivity impact on the organization. Lang (2009, 240) states that managerial time requirements for conflict issues have doubled since the 1980s, citing the reasons as "the growing complexity of organizations, use of teams and group decision making, and globalization." Furthermore, workplace conflict affects employee morale, interpersonal relations, and turnover and can lead to litigation—all of which decrease an organization's **productivity**.

**Productivity**
The level of output related to input.

As implied earlier, conflict is an inevitable and even necessary reality in the workplace, whether caused by task-related issues, unclear policies, poor communication, or incompatible personalities of members assigned to the same workgroup. Differing opinions, values, goals, and priorities can trigger conflict as well, as conflict is a natural consequence of stressful workplace interactions combined with the complexities of human personalities. Conflict does not just go away on its own, and managers who ignore workplace conflicts only exacerbate the problem. As healthcare systems continue to grow and become increasingly intricate, conflict is possible at any time, and at any level of the organization.

The responsibilities of a managerial position require those in authority to achieve more than the target revenue numbers or to exceed stated goals. Dealing with conflict is one of the toughest challenges managers face, and it is often a skill area in which managers feel less than prepared. At times, managers must successfully function as a counselor, mediator, or negotiator to assist employees in resolving work-related disagreements. Some conflicts may be resolved using common sense, while others require a higher level of tact and skill, as some conflicts have legal consequences.

Therefore, managerial preparedness to handle conflict properly is critical. Correctly managing conflict and channeling it in a positive way can not only avert productivity and other workplace issues but also be beneficial to the organization in the long run by bringing about improvement and change. In light of the importance of this managerial responsibility, this chapter discusses workplace conflict, its causes, the different managerial styles used to address it, specific strategies for conflict resolution, and tips on preventing conflict.

## The Nature of Conflict in the Workplace

Conflict may spike quickly or emerge slowly over time and in several ways. First, conflict may develop within an individual, as in someone who feels torn between what she wants to do and what she is expected to do. These internal conflicts may be ethical, such that the individual faces a dilemma that presents two or more paths of decision making.

Second, conflict may occur between two employees for a variety of reasons, some of which are discussed later. In these situations of **interpersonal conflict**, one or more of the conflicting parties may be described as "difficult to work with," perhaps because they are perceived to behave in ways that are at odds with prevailing values or stances regarding the issues at hand. Conflict between two employees may be resolved directly or indirectly in time, through managerial intervention, employee attrition, or assigned positional changes, or it may persist for years, having a lasting impact on communication, decision making, and overall productivity.

**Interpersonal conflict**
Discord between two or more individuals.

Third, conflict is seen whenever employees are required to work collaboratively on teams and in workgroups. Amid conflict, some teams thrive and succeed, while others suffer a total breakdown and fail to be productive. Bradley and colleagues (2015) point out that as team-based tasks increase in the work environment, managers must have a solid understanding of the causes of the conflict and the impact it has on overall productivity.

Dealing with conflict successfully is a skill learned in part through observation, communication, and resolution efforts. To begin, managers must be familiar with the common causes of conflict in the workplace to be able to identify where conflict commonly starts.

## The Most Common Causes of Workplace Conflict

Conflict can take place any time a disagreement or opposition arises related to ideas, demands, wishes, or interests. Some of the causes of conflict reflect their source on the basis of beliefs, attitudes, or values. In addition, these causes may be either actual differences or perceived differences (of which the perception may or may not be correct and justified). Perception is a huge factor in the cause and perpetuation of conflict in the workplace. It can be the sole cause of conflict or add to the depth and strength of an emotional response to a real difference (van Servellen 2009).

Following is a list of causes of conflict frequently seen on the individual, group, and organizational level.

- *Differences in values.* Conflict over values often occurs when each person or group sees the situation from its own worldview only, which may not align with that of others. The variables of gender, cultural diversity, religion, education, stage of life, and professional experiences can strongly influence the emergence and direction of a conflict.
- *Disparate goals and personal interests.* If the employees or group members are overly focused on their own individual needs, goals, or objectives, the likelihood of conflict rises.
- *Personality clashes.* Sometimes, employees simply do not get along. The intricacies of the self and variances in personality types may cause conflict resulting from difficulties in interpersonal dialogue and disruption to the team environment.
- *Personal problems brought into the workplace.* Employees who are under a high level of stress at home may exhibit uncharacteristic behaviors in the workplace, which may lead coworkers to feel this stress is being taken out on them.
- *Poor work environment.* Some environments are shaped by policies, procedures, or managerial practices that are inadequate, unclear, or unfair. In healthcare, overlapping job responsibilities or unclear boundaries are common causes of a problematic work environment. Whether the difficulties have been inherited from an incompetent former manager or originated with a failing current manager, such conflict must be identified and assessed.
- *Professional rivalries.* Rivalries often emerge between individual employees, groups of employees, or entire departments. They can be healthy and lead to improved productivity, or they can be a means of intimidation requiring intervention.
- *Competition for limited resources.* As with rivalries, conflict over resources can occur between employees, groups of employees, or departments. Time is a significant resource at the core of many conflicts, which can affect not only the hospital or health system but also the entire healthcare sector in terms of staffing shortages, heavy workloads, and the need for long shifts.
- *Unrealistic due dates for special work assignments.* Staffs' regular workload combined with additional responsibilities can be a source of high pressure and tension, leading to one or more types of conflict.

- *Difficult times for the organization.* The stress of financial instability, reorganization, right-sizing, mergers, or new ventures can increase the chances of conflict (Brent and Dent 2014). Lack of or poor communication about operational viability feeds anxiety, rumors, and discord, especially in the absence of certainty that measures are being taken to address the difficulties and keep the organization running.

- *Disparities in knowledge, power, or position in the organizational hierarchy.* Such gaps are inherent in healthcare organizations, as the different levels of care providers often introduce clashes over patient care issues and decision making. As the number of hierarchical levels increase, the probability and intensity of conflict increase as well.

- *Interdependent tasks.* In cases where one employee cannot complete her work until other employees have completed theirs, significant stress and frustration can result, which begets interpersonal conflict as well as failure to reach team goals.

- *Rapid change in the environment.* A large amount of change in a short period can put some employees on edge, which may be a predisposing factor in conflict.

- *Ethical issues.* Ethics concerns may arise when managers or clinicians are pulled in two different directions by competing courses of action for a situation. This tension may arise from differing philosophies, inconsistent duties, or a poorly defined personal sense of right versus wrong. Add in the emotional dimension inherent in healthcare delivery, and one can see how ethical issues may lead to conflict and heated discussion.

- *Personal misunderstandings due to inadequate communication between employees.* Misunderstandings often are caused by an inability of one employee (or the leader of a workgroup) to clearly articulate his position or needs. Equally common is misunderstanding caused by poor listening skills.

Most parties in a workplace conflict spend the majority of their time talking instead of listening. While one employee is speaking, the other(s) may be thinking of a response that will support his viewpoint. Important information from the opposite side of the conflict is missed, and the opportunity to learn passes. This breakdown of active listening, which is common in healthcare environments, only deepens the conflict.

Additionally, most employees immediately judge the statements of others—quickly agreeing or disagreeing with the first point that is heard. This rush to judgment can stem from an aligned point of view that fails to consider the other employee's viewpoint or reasoning.

The impact of any conflict may be detrimental to both the individuals involved and the healthcare organization in which they work. Furthermore, any causes of conflict may deepen or worsen conflicts that already exist.

### The Role of Perception in Conflict

As explained earlier in the chapter, conflict is more than just a simple disagreement; it is a situation in which employees perceive a threat to their well-being. One key to understanding conflict, then, is to recognize the role of **perception** in these situations.

**Perception**
The way an individual views the world.

To many people, including employees, their perception is their reality, whether or not they are correct in their perception. Managers who have an awareness of how perception influences workplace conflict can respond appropriately to the conflict.

The following are just a few factors that may drive individuals' perceptions:

- *Gender.* Men and women tend to perceive situations differently on the basis of their life and workplace experiences. These perceptions may relate to status and hierarchical position as outward signs of power. The level of perceived power in the situation can lead to variations in the mind-set with which a conflict is approached.

- *Ethnicity, race, and culture.* From childhood, our upbringing and instilled values have taught us to hold certain beliefs about the social structure of the world around us. Part of this belief system is the importance of conflict and conflict avoidance in our lives. These influences can cause employees to demonstrate different physical and psychological responses to conflict, including aggressiveness, passivity, and different levels of willingness to engage in dialogue.

- *Previous experiences with conflict.* Although frequently unknown to the manager, some of her employees may have encountered significant, profound life experiences involving conflict that now affect their perception of any conflict situation. As a result, they may feel afraid, untrusting, and unwilling to take even small risks. They may display conflict-avoidant behavior, shying away from the unknown and lacking confidence in their roles.

- *Education.* Whether from formal or informal instruction, an employee's knowledge has a direct impact on his level of preparedness to engage in the conflict at hand. Those with a higher level of education tend to be more confident and outspoken, often with refined rhetoric skills that allow them to carry on strong—sometimes intimidating— conversations. In addition to formal education, less formal knowledge, such as that acquired on the job, affects one's perception of the conflict by potentially limiting one's willingness to accept alternatives. Situation-specific knowledge also affects the conflict management process (discussed in detail later) in a variety of ways.

## Common Emotional Responses to Conflict

Together, the aforementioned factors may be manifested in a negative attitude or in a positive, optimistic outlook, leading us to another dimension of conflict: emotional responses.

In addition to behavioral responses to conflict, a manager should expect employees to react on emotional, cognitive, and sometimes physical levels. For example, employees who are at odds over conflicting values and then asked to cooperate to find a solution may respond with anger or resentment. In this section, we highlight some important signs that can be observed in employees to help understand their experiences during and after a conflict and to provide clues about the true source of the perceived threat, which may provide additional insight into a situation.

**Physiological responses** to conflict are straightforward to identify. Managers should look for signs of heightened stress, such as increased perspiration, muscle tension, shallow or accelerated breathing, or paleness that might signal nausea.

**Cognitive responses**, though present, are not easy to observe. They comprise the internal dialogue one has with oneself during an interaction. Cognitive responses may be evident as an appearance of distraction or distance during a conversation or meeting.

Emotional responses are the most readily attributable reactions to conflict. Is a normally outspoken employee now quiet, or is a quiet employee now outspoken? Outward behavioral expressions of conflict may range from the primary emotion of anger to one or more of the secondary emotions of confusion and hurt that underlie the anger, as well as a sense of loss of control over the outcome of the conflict or another complex emotional reaction.

In the heat of the moment, a manager may have difficulty sorting through all of these behavioral and cognitive responses of the parties involved, let alone prioritizing those that most need attention. The caution here is that a manager responding to only one emotion (e.g., anger) may lead the employee to suppress other feelings (e.g., confusion, disappointment). Although appropriate to appreciate all the emotions present, it is nearly impossible to respond to each one. Managers can prioritize them to the best of their ability and take note of other feelings to address later, when the opportunity arises for a one-on-one meeting.

A manager may be reluctant to deal with employees' emotions, but successful leaders do so when necessary to manage conflict. If employees embroiled in a conflict show multiple signs of stress or anger, one course

**Physiological response**
An automatic, instinctive response to a stressful situation manifesting in observable physical markers such as heightened blood pressure, heart rate, muscle tension, and a change in breathing patterns.

**Cognitive response**
The set of thoughts or silent personal self-talk that occurs during an interaction.

of action is to meet with them one-on-one and allow them to vent their concerns. The process of venting tends to lower stress-mediated responses and may bring the parties to a calm and productive mind-set from which to approach their work. Strategies for addressing conflict are presented in detail later in the Conflict Management section of this chapter.

## The High Cost of Conflict in Healthcare Organizations

Carefully observe the emotions you see in your employees when conflict is present or brewing. Do you see any verbal or nonverbal cues, such as indicators of anger, fear, disappointment, confusion, sadness, guilt, or frustration over the situation? Do you hear any inappropriate or off-handed comments, verbal attacks, or defensive responses? Have you noted any exaggerated facial expressions, or witnessed (or heard about) attempts at backstabbing or manipulation? These types of actions and reactions are often confusing and hurtful to the receiving party and have the potential to poison the larger work environment.

The costs and consequences of conflict in the healthcare workplace are numerous and can have a staggeringly negative impact on the organization if not handled properly and in a timely manner. As you read this section of the chapter, keep in mind that you are, or someday will be, managing an organization that has a *direct impact on patients' lives*—a serious undertaking. Whether a pair of clinicians arguing over the dimensions of care or two departments haggling over budget cost centers, most conflicts lead to a loss of productivity at a minimum and may result in patient harm or litigation.

In their book *Becoming a Conflict Competent Leader*, Runde and Flanagan (2013, 17) explain that "when conflict is mismanaged, costs mount. Some out-of-pocket costs like absenteeism and lawsuits are relatively easy to see and compute. Others, like poor decision-making, lost opportunities and diminished quality of working relationships, can prove more costly, but they are more difficult to quantify." They offer seven points of consideration to help illustrate the high cost of conflict in an organization.

### Point 1. The Amount of Wasted Time for Manager and Employee
How much time is spent on the conflict rather than focused on productive activity that directly improves patient care, helps the organization reach goals, or adds to the financial stability of the organization? Monitoring a tense environment, holding extra meetings, and actively resolving medium- or high-level conflict can be a time-consuming process, quickly taking up most of a morning or an afternoon, for example. Soon, this time expenditure has pushed a large portion of both the manager's and employees' duties to

the side, forcing them to catch up in the time that remains. In addition to productivity time, factor in idle time of employees or managers who stop to complain or gossip to their coworkers or colleagues about the conflict. When staff are rushed to complete their tasks, patient care and other matters can suffer in terms of quality.

### Point 2. Employee Turnover

When conflict in the workplace is ongoing, many employees seek a better and calmer place of employment. Runde and Flanagan (2013, 18) note that "the replacement cost of finding, training, and bringing a new person up to speed can often exceed the annual salary of the employee who leaves. It certainly costs more than addressing conflicts in the first place so employees do not get frustrated and leave. If turnover becomes an organizational problem, an effective leader needs to determine if poorly managed conflict is at least partially at fault." Employee turnover due to conflict is a serious leadership pitfall, as many good employees are lost because conflict is left unchecked.

### Point 3. Complaints, Grievances, and Lawsuits

If conflict can be spotted and addressed quickly and the potential damage limited, the overall cost of the experience is lower than if its handling is delayed or inadequate. In addition, when conflict is ignored, it may spiral out of control and require much more time and a higher level of intervention, which requires more effort and cost to the organization. One estimate cites the cost and time impact at $50,000 to $100,000 per incident and three to five years' average time frame to settle an incident (Mihm and Fairbank 2012). These types of expenditures represent money and effort that could have been used to improve processes or engage in other opportunities.

### Point 4. Employee Absenteeism and Healthcare Costs

In cases of conflict that are particularly stressful or unpleasant for those involved, employees may either stay home from work or leave work early to avoid dealing with it. Not only does their time away cost the organization in terms of lost productivity, but also these employees tend to seek out medical services to assist them in dealing with stress-related illnesses, which adds to the cost of the organization's healthcare insurance. Depending on the positions of the employees, additional part-time or substitute workers may need to be called in and paid to replace those who are taking time off for this reason—often at the last minute.

### Point 5. Violence in the Workplace

Conflict can become physical, which requires the assistance of security personnel or the local police department. Runde and Flanagan (2013, 19) caution that "A significant number of these assaults come from disgruntled customers, patients, coworkers and employees. The emotional toll on the targets of the violence as well as on their coworkers can be enormous and can increase the costs associated with retention, absenteeism and healthcare." In addition, consider that the aggressor in a physical assault in the workplace is typically fired immediately, leading to the expense of replacing him or her. The violence may also lead to litigation, which makes violence a multifaceted problem for managers to handle.

### Point 6. Errors and Poor Decision Making

The stress, distraction, and disruption of conflict hinder the ability of employees or managers to function with a clear and relaxed mind, which can affect decision making. Energy in the work setting becomes lowered, creativity is lost, and errors occur. Employees resist presenting new ideas, hesitate to communicate with others for fear of further conflict, and are unwilling to take risks. Considered together, these factors lower the quality of decision making. To illustrate, Rowe and Sherlock (2005, 245) surveyed 213 nurses and found that 13 percent of them stated that being involved "in verbally heated conflicts" led them to "make a caregiving error." In addition, Haraway and Haraway (2005, 12) found that nearly every healthcare worker "can recall delays or inadequacies in patient care caused by a provider refusing to consult the 'on call' physician or group for a problem outside of their area of expertise because of some unresolved past conflict."

### Point 7. A Poisoned Relationship Workplace

Conflict often comes with a wide variety of unpleasant emotions, including anger, embarrassment, hurt, fear, frustration, guilt, loss of control, defensiveness, and distrust. Negativity in the workplace is toxic to all who are exposed to it, and morale decreases as a result. No one wants to come to work to experience these feelings.

## Conflict Management

Conflict management is the process of actively limiting the negative effects of conflict while allowing positive discussion and challenging interactions to take place. In conflict management, the goal is to enhance every party's understanding of the issue by facilitating calm and helpful discussions on the main points of disagreement. This understanding allows for rational dialogue; the presentation and consideration of options; and, in most cases, an effective outcome. If conflict is properly managed, the learning opportunities and discourse it generates can be channeled to improve the outcomes of the workgroup because of the intellectual challenge and the high level of group involvement (Alper, Tjosvold, and Law 2000).

Highly effective conflict management should produce the following results (Ledlow and Coppola 2014, 121):

- A wise agreement, if an agreement is possible
- An efficient solution
- A potentially innovative solution
- Movement toward positive change in the organization
- A better relationship between the conflicting parties, or at least no damage to the relationship

In light of these expectations, how should healthcare managers best address conflict? A good place to start is to realize that different conflicts require different conflict management styles and approaches. Not only should healthcare managers be trained in handling conflict but all important stakeholders should receive specific training on effectively handling conflict as well.

**Primary conflict tension**, or the stress of the initial conflict, is usually followed by secondary conflict tension triggered by the process of dealing with the conflict as it plays out over time. Both require healthcare managers to intervene quickly to handle the conflict and thus limit the amount of negative consequences that may result. Without intervention, employees may get stuck in negativity and unproductiveness and suffer from damaged relationships. If a conflict persists, the manager is responsible for monitoring the work environment for the factors noted in this chapter, as time carries its own impact on conflict as well.

> **Primary conflict tension**
> The stress produced by the initial conflict.

Depending on how a manager handles the conflicts that arise in her area, employees either come to welcome her as a leader or become wary of dealing with her if they learn she is unable to resolve difficult situations. Conflict management can ultimately affect a manager's reputation and career, so she must be prepared to actively assist with or intervene in the conflict at any time to keep her employees and teams working well. This preparedness begins with the clear understanding of one's personal conflict management style.

## Understanding Your Conflict Management Style

Even if you have not held a managerial position yet, you have a **conflict management style**. To discover how you manage conflict, over the next few weeks, note how you typically handle conflict and interpersonal tensions in your personal and professional life. Think about the causes of the conflicts, the process used in resolving them, and the outcomes of the conflicts.

> **Conflict management style**
> The way a leader handles situations of discord.

After a few conflicts have occurred, pause to reflect on them in terms of the following questions:

- Do you notice a pattern to the conflicts?
- How do you describe yourself in a conflict situation?
- Are you withdrawn, avoiding the situation and hoping it will pass if you ignore it long enough?
- Are you a readily agreeable peacemaker, allowing the other party to "win" and have their way?
- Are you generally disagreeable or aggressive in nature, working toward the classic win–lose outcome?
- Are you constructive, encouraging collaboration and discussion before an outcome is reached for the good of the situation?
- How often are the outcomes of your conflicts satisfactory, and how often do negative results, hurt feelings, or damaged relationships occur as part of the outcome?

On the basis of this simple analysis, decide whether you would like to change your conflict management style. If you do want to make some changes, develop a plan of action to achieve them. Many excellent resources are available, including textbooks, websites, and conferences, as well as conversations with colleagues and mentors who can provide ideas and suggestions (Davis et al. 1996).

After you reflect and make any changes that you desire, repeat this analysis on the next few conflicts that occur in your life. How did the new results compare with the first round of results? Were you able to reach more satisfactory agreements?

Every individual has a dominant or primary style of resolving conflict, as well as a secondary style. Just as the typical day-to-day aspects of personality tend to be consistent, so does a manager's approach to handling conflicts in the workplace. Consistency in the personal qualities displayed is important, as it is in one's method of addressing conflict when it arises. Therefore, a crucial step in this area of leadership is twofold: Review and consider the ways in which conflict can be resolved, and choose one that suits your personality and setting of use as the primary means to deal with it. Once you have arrived at the go-to method and have had some experience handling conflict, you may also adopt a secondary or contingency style of conflict management. The discussion of conflict management strategies that follows highlights strategies to consider.

## Conflict Management Strategies

A variety of conflict management strategies can be learned in a short amount of time and mastered over the long term (Ledlow and Coppola 2014). The more time a manager spends learning and practicing the seven strategies presented here, the more flexible and prepared he will be when these skills are needed in actual conflict situations.

### Forcing

The forcing style relies on the formal power inherent in managerial positions to end the conflict. It is an authoritative style that does not work well in all situations yet is sometimes necessary, as in the case of severe time constraints.

In the forcing strategy, the situation is decided single-handedly and quickly. The potential downside of this strategy is that it often does not adequately consider the concerns of those on both sides of the conflict. Therefore, if this strategy is used, the manager should recognize that he must first listen to the points made by all involved and then render a final decision. Depending on the outcome, all will not be pleased with the result, and the leader may need to take steps to enhance the understanding of those on the "losing" side and subsequently repair relationships with those involved.

### Accommodating

The leader using the accommodating style agrees to allow those on one side of the conflict to have their way while those on the other side concede their original position or proposal in the conflict. This strategy may seem to constitute simply giving in to the one side over the concerns of the other, and indeed that may be all that is involved in certain situations, as when one side is indisputably correct. Over time, your experience may inform these decisions. When this style is applied, the accommodation should be explained with care to employees.

At other times, more information may be needed about both positions before a judgment accommodating one side over the other can be made. In these cases, the manager leads a discussion in which both sides further explain any unclear points. Allowing a small passage of time before holding this meeting may decrease the intensity of the emotion, clearing space for everyone involved to reflect on what the perceived opponent is saying. You may determine that one proposal is indeed feasible as is, or (more likely), you may find it is workable with additional constructive group communication to resolve the point of conflict.

Accommodating is a desirable strategy to choose if the conflict is over a noncritical issue or, as mentioned earlier, if the manager realizes in the midst of the conflict that one party is clearly wrong. The conflict can then be resolved quickly and amicably without risking damage to the opposing parties' working relationship. Furthermore, it may build social capital or goodwill that can be used later to address other issues.

## Avoiding

Some managers deal with conflict by actively or passively avoiding it; they choose not to take any visible actions to resolve it. Although some conflicts may die out in time, many worsen to the point that emotions take over and the working relationships of the employees involved are permanently changed or severed. Brent and Dent (2014) note that although this is the preferred strategy of some leaders, it rarely makes the conflict stop or go away. It simply pushes the conflict aside for a short period.

Avoiding should be reserved for situations in which the issue is insignificant or when waiting a short time before resolving the conflict carries a clear advantage, such as the need to pause to gather more information or verify relevant facts. However, the leader should recognize that she may be putting personal relationships at risk by waiting.

The avoiding style can also be a helpful strategy if a cooling-off period is needed between parties, allowing a calm perspective to return. In this case, a defined period is announced (e.g., after lunch, tomorrow, Monday morning) to make all aware that the resolution is only temporarily tabled.

## Compromising

The compromising style, or meeting in the middle ground by partially pleasing both parties, usually quells a conflict. But leaders should understand that in a compromise, neither side completely gets its way. Each must give up some portion of its stance to allow the resolution to occur.

Although this style is often effective, leaders should monitor the parties following a compromise decision for unresolved feelings among those who are ill-equipped to handle adversity.

## Collaborating

In the collaborating style, both parties must be open to listening carefully and learning from each other to find a mutually satisfying solution that both sides find not only acceptable but also pleasing. Open discussion is key, as is a positive outlook on the situation. The sides must want to work together to find the best possible collaborative solution.

When using this strategy, leaders should carefully determine the amount of control they exercise over the group during the discussions, as exhibiting a high level of managerial control can dissuade some employees from speaking up or asking questions that may be beneficial to the resolution. Managers should lead the employees in a discussion that aims to find an integrative solution, encouraging all to share their thoughts and ideas, then merge the insights that are contributed to the resolution.

## Competing

The competing strategy can be used when a quick and decisive solution must be found, such as in an emergency or when production needs to increase quickly. The key to this style of conflict management is the ability to appeal to the competitive spirit that lives in most employees. How much can they raise the bar in a difficult situation to improve the organization? How many more patients can be served in a safe and effective way to allow all to receive the care they need when demand for services is high? How many days can each area go without a safety incident or patient complaint? Turning the issue into a supervised competition can help in situations involving unpopular actions that must be taken, such as cost cutting (Ledlow and Coppola 2014).

## Problem Solving

The problem-solving approach only works if both sides of the conflict agree to use it. If the problem is not personnel related but rather is an organizational issue, this strategy is an option. The problem can be presented to a specific workgroup, studied well by all stakeholders, and examined carefully before the workgroup chooses the solution to end the conflict.

Whether the conflict is a personal or professional one, leaders tend to use only one or two of the strategies presented here. For example, one may choose to collaborate when dealing with an interpersonal conflict, which carries the advantages that come with creative problem solving and idea sharing. But collaboration can be time consuming, so if time is a factor in the conflict, another strategy must be chosen. The most skilled managers learn to quickly assess the conflict and the associated level of emotion and then choose the most appropriate management strategy to match the type of conflict and surrounding factors.

## *Moderating Conflict*

Moderating conflict can be among the most challenging aspects of the managerial role. Leaders who have difficulty keeping their footing in the middle of a conflict may benefit from the following tips:

- Focus on the specific conflict only, not on related issues. Redirect the employees to the issue at hand if the conversation gets off track.
- Concentrate on positivity, leading by example. Negativity ruins the process before it begins.
- Separate people from the problem as much as possible. If small teams must negotiate the outcome of a conflict, choose participants with good self-control and neutral personalities rather than those who tend to be outspoken or are known to clash with each other. This approach

to participant selection keeps a professional focus on the problem itself, rather than possibly setting up a situation in which aspects of personality exacerbate the problem.

- Ask those who are outwardly emotional or exceedingly negative to leave the room until they are calm enough to participate in a positive way.
- Encourage the generation of as many ideas as possible before the final decision is made.
- Frequently ask if all involved in the conflict have had the chance to present their thoughts to the extent they wish to.
- Ask the group to think about the best and worst solutions. What are you (or the group) able to accept or not accept?
- Remind the group of the ramifications of the conflict being unsolved. This approach helps unify the parties to deliver a positive outcome for the department or organization.
- Call for a break for the whole group if emotions escalate. A time-out allows the tension to dissipate and can help the parties regain composure and perspective.
- Involve a neutral third party or professional mediator. This solution brings added expense, but the cost of the conflict to the organization may be higher in the long run.

### Choosing a Conflict Management Strategy

To most effectively resolve a workplace conflict, leaders should aim to use the strategy that is most appropriate for that situation. However, that strategy might not be the manager's preferred style, or she may be part of the conflict.

Understanding one's role in the situation is important as the process begins. The leader should consider all the surrounding factors of the conflict, including time, severity, and emotions. We recommend the following steps in preparing to handle a workplace conflict:

- Carefully and logically select the strategy to use, and be clear—for yourself and to others—on why this strategy will work the best as opposed to the other options in that situation.
- Rehearse the strategy, and be prepared with factual documentation if necessary to discuss the situation with confidence.
- Stay calm and level-headed. A manager who is personally involved in the conflict should walk away briefly if tensions rise. Focus on being as objective as possible.
- Act professionally and avoid making judgments. Be wary of non-fact-based information, such as rumors or unproven statements.

- Let the employees vent their anger in a constructive way. Part of the anger often comes from the parties feeling they have not been heard. Once it has been expressed, set the anger aside and focus on the issue behind the conflict only.
- Do not ignore how you feel about the process, and be clear about what you want or need from the resolution.
- Consider how others feel, as well as what they want and need. Understand that emotions can affect behaviors in uncharacteristic ways. Try to put yourself in their situation, and take whatever steps are feasible to defuse the tension.
- Know ahead of time the resource implications and other limitations of each potential solution to the conflict.
- Stay prepared to change your approach if the situation warrants.

Several factors that must be considered when choosing a conflict management strategy include the manager's interpersonal relationship with those on the opposite side of the conflict (if relevant), the resources available, the resources that cannot be obtained, the amount of time available to resolve the conflict, and the importance of the issues at hand. Ledlow and Coppola (2014, 124) suggest that leaders ask themselves the following questions as part of their strategic decision-making process in conflict management:

- Is (are) the issue (issues) important to you?
- Is (are) the issue (issues) important to the other party?
- Is the relationship with the other party important to you?
- How much time is available and how much pressure/stress is there to come to resolution?
- How much do you trust the other party?

The best strategy to use depends on the individual conflict situation, so matching the style to the conflict should be carefully undertaken. However, leaders must be aware that the party on one side of the conflict may choose one strategy while the opposite side (knowingly or not) may choose a different strategy. This scenario makes communication even more vital as the resolution process plays out so that as many roadblocks as possible are removed.

## Anticipating and Preventing Conflict in the Workplace

Prevention of conflict is worth the time and effort it takes to avoid having to manage and resolve conflict after it happens. To that end, following are specific steps toward preventing conflict among individuals or groups of employees:

- *State that professionalism and respect are expectations in the workplace.* Right from the start, be open and firm about this expectation. If you notice the start of a personality-related conflict, advise (or remind) all to interact professionally and appropriately.
- *Assign clear roles.* Ambiguity in roles leads to conflict as well as ineffectiveness. Be clear in what each team member is expected to contribute to the good of the workgroup. Put this information in writing, and share it with all involved to eliminate potential confusion.
- *Build a sense of teamwork in your setting.* Emphasize the "we" from the beginning of the group's formation, and use team-based goal setting and incentives to achieve cohesion.
- *Be cautious with difficult decision making.* Tough decision making and decision announcement are potential areas of conflict. When difficult decisions must be made, how do you approach them? Have all the facts been gathered, points been clarified, and time taken to consider the alternatives as well as short- and long-term consequences of the decision? Are you in a calm mood that lends itself to sound decision making? If not, refrain from stating your decision until the tension of the conflict passes (Healey and Marchese 2012).
- *Make sure resource allocations among team members are fair.* This equality prevents the "more than, less than" type of arguments that can be the source of conflict.
- *Try to minimize the growth of smaller intragroup cliques.* Try assigning small group sizes early on. In most cases, two to four people per workgroup is best to prevent clique development. The greater number of people assigned to the workgroup, the greater the potential for conflict.
- *Request that all workgroup discussions take place in the confines of the group.* Sidebar or behind-the-back conversations—whether verbal or via e-mail—often breed tension and conflict, so these discussions must be discouraged. All team members should be copied on all communications (Dye and Garman 2015). Provide opportunities for all participants to discuss the group's goals, processes, difficulties, accomplishments, and so on in an open and (if needed) moderated forum.
- *Take care to not assign incompatible personalities to the same workgroup.* If you put time into getting to know key employees and team leaders, you can observe their personality traits in a relatively short time.

- *In workgroups, state that you expect decision making by consensus only.* One or two employees may not rule by dictating.

- *Assign a reasonable timeline for the work to be completed,* with fair due dates on each portion to be accomplished. Heightened time constraints and related anxiety trigger the potential for conflict.

- *Anticipate seasonal changes in the workload that raise stress and predispose conflict.* What preparations can be made to anticipate this occurrence? One option is to assign larger projects in the slow times of the year.

- *Provide an open channel for employees to report problems and concerns with their workgroups* before they result in full-blown conflict. Dealing with problems while they are small is easier than letting them grow into larger, more significant and costly ones.

As a final comment on anticipating conflict in the workplace, be aware that when ethical principles are involved, as is common in the healthcare environment, the outcome is likely to cause a conflict. With many stakeholders present in the healthcare system—managers, care providers, individual patients, families of patients, and the community—clashes in values are not uncommon. In fact, many hospital accreditation bodies and government regulators now require ethical values to be consistently examined, monitored, and addressed, especially in the areas of physician integrity, confidentiality of information, conflicts of interest, and research ethics. A significant responsibility of healthcare leaders is to create, and then orient all staff to, an ethical climate that is consistent with the mission of the organization and the expectations of employees and patients.

The ethical conflicts that arise during one's managerial career are not always straightforward—sometimes the gray area is deep and distressing. Leaders must not only be educated in but also stay up-to-date on the discipline of ethics so that the ethical climate is relevant to the times and well understood by all. This effort allows the development of a clear, preventive process to resolve any ethics-based conflicts or tensions that arise (Healey and Marchese 2012).

## The Energizing Influence of Conflict on Teams

Conflict in workplace teams can occasionally be a source of renewed energy, which has the potential to bring about a positive result. Managers or team leaders who constructively challenge each other's thinking develop an enhanced and complete understanding of the decision-making options available. Specifically, conflict can be energizing because it does the following:

- *Ends complacency.* Challenge allows employees to shift from the routine of being satisfied with everything to being concerned about everything. They start to question the status quo, including (possibly ineffective) practices, policies, traditions, and decisions.
- *Initiates discussion.* An eerie silence may ensue as conflict is brewing and the involved parties begin to strategize their next move, but discussion soon ignites as the conflict progresses and deepens. These discussions, when properly managed and moderated, can bring about breakthrough resolution.
- *Steers action.* Even if the action is not optimal or feasible in a given situation, conflict inspires action rather than inaction.
- *Demands participation.* Employees who are otherwise silent and reserved typically become involved as a conflict becomes apparent, especially if encouraged to do so. Their views on the situation may need to be shared, or sides may need to be taken. At times, the best solutions emerge from the quietest employees—who are often the best listeners.

## Summary

When intelligent, opinionated people come together, conflict is bound to arise. Encourage openness in all discussions, and be sure that all ideas and concerns are voiced before a final decision is made. Do not be afraid to intervene in a conflict. If it progresses too far, time is wasted, outcomes deteriorate, the working relationships of the employees involved are perhaps permanently damaged, and litigation becomes possible. With such potentially high prices for the organization and its employees to pay, it is up to you to lead your setting well and keep conflict to a minimum.

## Discussion Questions

1. How does communication affect conflict?
2. What are some of the most common causes of conflict in the workplace?
3. Describe your personal conflict management style. How can this be a good or bad approach in the managerial setting?
4. What are some costs of conflict to healthcare organizations?
5. What are the seven conflict management strategies? Describe a situation in which each would be helpful to bring about a resolution.
6. As a manager, how can you work to prevent conflict in your work setting?

# References

Alper, S., D. Tjosvold, and K. S. Law. 2000. "Conflict Management, Efficacy, and Performance in Organizational Teams." *Personnel Psychology* 53: 625–42.

Bradley, B. H., H. J. Anderson, J. E. Baur, and A. C. Klotz. 2015. "When Conflict Helps: Integrating Evidence for Beneficial Conflict in Groups and Teams Under Three Perspectives." *Group Dynamics: Theory, Research, and Practice* 19 (4): 243–72.

Brent, M., and F. E. Dent. 2014. *The Leader's Guide to Managing People: How to Use Soft Skills to Get Hard Results.* New York: Pearson.

Davis, B. L., C. J. Skube, L. W. Hellervik, S. H. Gebelein, and J. L. Sheard. 1996. *Successful Manager's Handbook: Development Suggestions for Today's Managers.* Minneapolis, MN: PDI Ninth House.

Dye, C. F., and A. N. Garman. 2015. *Exceptional Leadership: 16 Critical Competencies for Healthcare Executives.* Chicago: Health Administration Press.

Haraway, D. L., and W. M. Haraway III. 2005. "Analysis of the Effect of Conflict-Management and Resolution Training on Employee Stress at a Health Care Organization." *Hospital Topics* 83 (4): 11–17.

Healey, B. J., and M. Marchese. 2012. *Foundations of Health Care Management: Principles and Methods.* San Francisco: Jossey-Bass.

Lang, M. 2009. "Conflict Management: A Gap in Business Education Curricula." *Journal of Education for Business* 84 (4): 240–45.

Ledlow, G. R., and M. N. Coppola. 2014. *Leadership for Health Professionals: Theory, Skills and Applications.* Burlington, MA: Jones & Bartlett Learning.

Mihm, D., and M. Fairbank. 2012. "Workplace Conflict and Your Business." Dispute Resolution Center of Yakima and Kittitas Counties. Accessed February 17, 2017. http://c.ymcdn.com/sites/nafcm.site-ym.com/resource/resmgr/Research/Workplace_Conflict_and_Your_.pdf.

Rowe, M., and H. Sherlock. 2005. "Stress and Verbal Abuse in Nursing: Do Burned Out Nurses Eat Their Young?" *Journal of Nursing Management* 13 (3): 242–48.

Runde, C. E., and T. A. Flanagan. 2013. *Becoming a Conflict Competent Leader: How You and Your Organization Can Manage Conflict Effectively.* San Francisco: Jossey-Bass.

van Servellen, G. 2009. *Communication Skills for the Health Care Professional: Concepts, Practice, and Evidence.* Sudbury, MA: Jones & Bartlett.

# DEVELOPING LEADERS AND IMPROVING TEAM PERFORMANCE IN HEALTHCARE ORGANIZATIONS

Bernard J. Healey

## Learning Objectives

After completing this chapter, the reader should be able to

- describe the need for leadership in healthcare organizations,
- be capable of understanding the need for leadership development programs in healthcare organizations,
- explain the different methods used in leadership development in healthcare delivery, and
- discuss the value of completing a needs assessment for leadership training in a healthcare organization.

## Key Terms and Concepts

- Charismatic skills
- Internship
- Learning organization
- Management development
- Needs assessment
- Organizational life cycle
- Performance standard
- Self-efficacy

## Introduction

The overarching goal of this textbook is to help the providers of healthcare services offer consumers the best care possible. Throughout this book, mentioned time and again is the fact that a pressing need exists to reduce the cost of healthcare delivery while simultaneously improving the quality of the health services delivered. The overriding hypothesis is that one of the best ways to improve healthcare delivery is through strong leadership working with empowered followers. It also emphasizes that all followers in healthcare delivery roles should receive leadership training shortly after beginning their employment in a healthcare facility or program. They are all members of a team responsible for the improvement of services in their organization.

In addition, this text argues that leaders are not necessarily born but can be made through leadership development programs designed for future leaders. Therefore, healthcare organizations are called on to develop and implement a leadership training and development program for most, if not all, of their staff members. To begin this effort, the established leaders need to review all the available literature on what types of training yield the greatest success in the development of healthcare leaders.

Clearly, some organizations outperform others in the same industry while facing the same or similar challenges. These successful organizations are identified as having strong leadership, happy and dedicated employees, a strong purpose and values, and a thick positive culture. The competition attempts to duplicate these ingredients and, more often than not, fails in the attempt. This failure is attributed to the lack of a so-called super leader in the duplicating organizations, which is a hallmark of successful entities. Those organizations that have researched the benefits of strong leadership development and training programs realize that mere duplication is ineffective. Instead, they offer their staff training in leadership topics similar to successful organizations, followed by a rigorous evaluation process. This type of leadership training requires offering the right people the right training components delivered by the right instructor. This chapter focuses on the development of superior leadership training and team development programs for healthcare organizations.

## Exemplary Leadership Development Programs: Setting the Stage

According to Elsner and Farrands (2006), the vast majority of leaders are at a tremendous disadvantage when they begin their first leadership position because they know little about the people and culture of the businesses they are expected to lead. To overcome this challenge, the new leader must reach out to others in the company at the beginning part of the leadership transition to learn the culture and become familiar with the people in it as quickly as possible.

Once she has gained a foothold in understanding these aspects of her role, what does this leader need to learn next to succeed? And how does she gain that requisite knowledge and the appropriate experience? The answers to these questions form the basis for an organization to institute a leadership training and development program.

At the outset of creating such a program, healthcare organizations learn the differences between management development programs and leadership development programs. Bolden and colleagues (2011) point out that **management development** constitutes the provision of knowledge acquisition, skills training, and the nurturing of abilities to help managers improve their performance on current tasks. Leadership development, on the other hand, is the improvement of the individual's knowledge, skills, and abilities in anticipation of unknown challenges. This definition implies that by preparing people for the future, organizations also view leadership development as effective systems design.

**Management development**
Training programs that assist managers in job improvement.

Once the organization has gained a solid understanding of the differences between management training and leadership training, it should make the commitment to become a **learning organization**. In addition to the points made about learning organizations elsewhere in this book, Samit (2015) suggests that lifelong learning for employees is no longer a luxury but instead is mandatory for ensuring the long-term viability of the organization and the fulfillment of its employees. When considered in terms of the advances in technology made in the past year alone, it becomes clear how today's knowledge becomes obsolete by tomorrow.

**Learning organization**
An entity that places great value on the constant growth of employees in terms of education and training.

One caveat to relying on a program of lifelong learning as part of a robust leadership development initiative has to do with employees' readiness, willingness, and ability to acquire new skills to deal with rapid change. Not all employees are at the same level of acceptance and capability, for a number of reasons, and care should be taken to not assume they are. One reason relates to the concept of **self-efficacy**. Self-efficacy was described by Albert Bandura (1976), a renowned psychologist, as the belief or lack of belief that one can accomplish a goal or succeed in an activity. The influence of self-efficacy can be seen in many organizations' efforts to implement electronic health record systems (EHRs). As healthcare organizations began adopting EHRs, they neglected to consider employees' sense of self-efficacy in meeting the challenge of entering important patient data into a computer system with which they had no previous familiarity. Employees' answer to the problem was to enter data into the system and maintain a hard copy of the same record, defeating the goal of efficiency improvement.

**Self-efficacy**
The belief of individuals in whether they can or cannot accomplish a goal or perform an activity.

Another aspect of a leadership development program, according to White and Griffith (2016), is a formal leadership succession plan. The succession plan is designed to replace, immediately and seamlessly, those who leave their leadership position. The purpose of succession planning is to identify potential leadership vacancies along with potential replacements while noting, and planning to meet, the successors' training needs. An example of a succession plan is shown as part of an overall leadership management program design in exhibit 10.1.

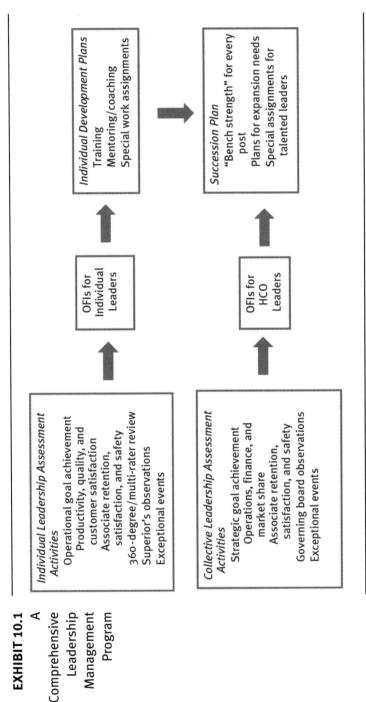

**EXHIBIT 10.1**

A Comprehensive Leadership Management Program

*Individual Leadership Assessment Activities*
Operational goal achievement
Productivity, quality, and customer satisfaction
Associate retention, satisfaction, and safety
360-degree/multi-rater review
Superior's observations
Exceptional events

*Collective Leadership Assessment Activities*
Strategic goal achievement
Operations, finance, and market share
Associate retention, satisfaction, and safety
Governing board observations
Exceptional events

OFIs for Individual Leaders

OFIs for HCO Leaders

*Individual Development Plans*
Training
Mentoring/coaching
Special work assignments

*Succession Plan*
"Bench strength" for every post
Plans for expansion needs
Special assignments for talented leaders

*Source:* White and Griffith (2016). HCO = healthcare organization; OFI = opportunity for improvement.

The program depicted in exhibit 10.1 highlights the important components of an exemplary leadership development and training program: leadership assessment activities; opportunities for improvement; individualized development plans; and, as discussed, a succession plan. Succession plans are valuable management tools for replacing key talent over time. They also signal to employees that internal promotion to leadership ranks is possible and may motivate staff to perform well. Finally, succession plans and accompanying training programs can drive a culture of excellence for the healthcare organization.

## What an Exemplary Leadership Development Program Looks Like

Employee training programs offer a systematic process to improve employees' capabilities with a goal of high performance and enhanced overall competence. All employees in healthcare organizations need to receive leadership training because they are all about to be empowered in their roles. To accept this empowerment requires gaining many of the skills and attributes of leadership and, therefore, should focus on moving employees in different directions than their old bureaucratic job description would allow. Exhibit 10.2 offers a general leadership development plan suitable for most types of employees of a healthcare organization. The plan calls for training to be completed in a short period and supplemented with real-world experiences at the facility.

Specifically, exhibit 10.2 is composed of a series of goals for the leadership development program, a set of topics to be covered through the learning experience, and a timeline for completion of each learning module. Nahavandi (2015) makes note of numerous content areas that can be addressed in a comprehensive leadership development program, and each organization should determine which components are relevant to its needs. These content areas include basic knowledge, personal growth information, skills development, creativity, and strategic issues related to the organization where the staff member works. As discussed in the remainder of this section, the leadership development plan starts with the needs assessment, moves to the key skills needed by the leader, and concludes with an evaluation process that determines the success or failure of the training and development program. The evaluation process also helps determine whether items should be added to or subtracted from the program.

The real key to success with leadership training and development programs is in both the qualifications of the instructors hired for the educational process and the motivation and engagement of the staff chosen to attend the programs.

**EXHIBIT 10.2**
Leadership
Development
Plan for
Healthcare
Organizations

| Goal of Training | Leadership Development Component | Time Frame |
|---|---|---|
| Assess needs | | |
| Establish specific leadership program objectives | | |
| Improve team leader-ship skills | | |
| Improve communication skills | | |
| Develop motivational and employee engage-ment skills | | |
| Develop intrapreneur-ship skills | | |
| Evaluate leadership development program | | |

### Employee Leadership Needs Assessment

The starting point for a leadership training and development program is an analysis of employee needs, referred to as a **needs assessment**. A needs assessment is a method for discovering, evaluating, and prioritizing what training is necessary to improve the performance of an employee in the organization. In recent years, the use of a needs assessment tool has become an important part of leadership training and development because it allows the organization to easily and inexpensively implement appropriate training for employees on the basis of the assessment findings. Furthermore, the assessment can be used to determine whether sufficient funds are available to provide training and budget for future training. Finally, it allows upper-level administrators to gauge leadership development needs in preparing staff for leadership assignments.

**Needs assessment**
A method of determining and prioritizing what individuals need to learn.

Once the needs for the leadership training are determined, the organization designs the training program. The design involves translating the needs of the leader candidate into specific objectives that become the outcome to be produced by the training process. The aim should be worded as a **performance standard** that can be measured at the end of the program and its accomplishment achieved in a certain amount of time.

**Performance standard**
A time-bound objective for an employee.

The next part of the needs assessment process identifies what must be learned to meet the objectives of the training program. Built into this portion of the needs assessment is a determination of how the individual candidate learns best.

## *Leadership Skills*

The most important skills for a leader in healthcare are team leadership, communication, motivational and employee engagement, culture-building, trust-building, and intrapreneurship skills.

### Team Leadership Skills

Team-based care comprises a large portion of healthcare services delivered to patients in many care settings. Thus, critical to understanding the nature of healthcare leadership in the twenty-first century is recognition that leadership is required not only at the top but throughout the entire organization. It follows that training these leaders requires a team-oriented focus. Presenting leadership training to all individuals in a healthcare organization brings numerous advantages, including the capacity to tap the collective genius fostered when a healthcare delivery team acts as one comprehensive unit.

Karlgaard and Malone (2015) have found that the highest-performing organizations exhibit the core strength of team excellence. The researchers reveal an important concept about teams that most people do not consider: When viewed as an organizational stucture, a team can also be seen as having an **organizational life cycle**. Over time, a team is formed, grows, reaches maturity, and eventually declines. The leader, therefore, must consider the life cycle of the team to see whether it needs to be refreshed with new members who may bring a renewed interest in the topic pursued by the team.

**Organizational life cycle**
The distinct stages of an organization's growth and decline.

Because teams in a learning organization receive the same leadership training and development as that provided to all the other leaders and followers in the healthcare organization, a key topic to be addressed is good followership. The skills required of leaders are similarly important for followers for the organization to meet the challenges faced now and in the future.

To solve the major problems in healthcare organizations discussed throughout this textbook, creativity and innovation are needed to guide the way healthcare services are developed and delivered. Contrary to popular wisdom, creativity and innovation do not have to come from the leaders in the organization; they can emerge from teams working together to solve problems. In fact, the team approach to organizational improvement through creativity and innovation has been shown to be far superior to the individual attempting to do it all. According to Hill and colleagues (2014), most leaders have been taught that they are responsible for coming up with the ideas and then convincing their followers to implement them. A much better policy is to have everyone on the team generate ideas because of the importance of collective wisdom to decision making. It coalesces the different bases of knowledge and experiences of team members who have been doing the work over time to make improvements.

According to White and Griffith (2016), one of the greatest strengths *and* weaknesses in healthcare delivery is the use of teams to provide patient care. They point to the great amount of patient information lost during a handoff from one team of caregivers to the next, causing mistakes and delays. These team errors are often the reason value is lost in the delivery of healthcare. The leader and team members must jointly determine enhanced ways to concentrate all team efforts on the patient receiving the care.

Karlgaard and Malone (2015, 20) argue that "the difference . . . between a perpetually successful enterprise and a struggling, dysfunctional also-ran comes down to the people in those enterprises and even more, to how those people relate to each other as they form and re-form into teams." Whenever patients are harmed by the healthcare process, inevitably a breakdown in communications has occurred. The way to eliminate the vast majority of never events is to instill team leadership qualities and knowledge in all team members, thereby improving the communication process among the teams delivering healthcare services.

## Communication Skills

One of the most important skills a leader must master is the ability to communicate effectively with employees and customers. To improve the quality of care delivered by healthcare facilities, a strong effort must be undertaken to keep everyone in the healthcare organization informed about the challenges faced and what is being done to meet these challenges. In fact, many health policy experts agree that better communications both inside and outside the organization can help the healthcare facility meet the demands of healthcare reform.

Few people are born with great communication skills. Those fortunate to have these skills are often thought to be natural leaders. However, these dual-ability individuals are the exception rather than the rule. Most experts in communication theory and development agree that to become a great communicator takes training, practice, and time to perfect the skill.

Communication skill is often taken for granted when one moves into a leadership position. This slight is a serious mistake to make because many managers and leaders in healthcare organizations are poor communicators, often because they have focused on honing other skills or have not been given the opportunity to learn the value of good communication skills.

According to Becker and Wortman (2009), companies that succeed have created a culture of communication in the workplace. That culture includes screening for communication ability in the interview process. This skill is so important that many organizations establish periodic communication training programs provided to all staff; this type of hardwiring can only take place when top leadership understands the value of communication, practices good communication styles themselves, and demands that everyone in the organization make a continuous effort to improve communications among all employees and leaders at all levels.

Many successful healthcare organizations have realized that rapid communications from top to bottom can result in numerous successful innovations. A well-developed communication system is also associated with enhanced employee engagement. As stated in chapter 9, much of the communication process in a well-run organization is founded in the ability of the leaders to listen as well as talk.

Another aspect of leadership communication is the concept of charisma. Nahavandi (2015) stresses the fact that leaders gain much by learning **charismatic skills**. He notes that charisma is instrumental in the development of an intense emotional bond between the leader and her followers. In addition, charismatic leaders are able to develop loyalty, motivate high performance, and inspire obedience when necessary through the use of their charismatic communication skills (Nahavandi 2015). Thus, any leadership development program needs to make charisma a key component of its approach for all employees. This characteristic is important for employees who deliver healthcare services to shape their interactions positively with other employees and customers on a daily basis.

**Charismatic skill**
Attractiveness and charm that can lead to devotion by others.

Times of crisis usually bring forth informal leaders who have gained power over others because they have learned the skill of charismatic communications. Even though they have no appointed power, they have gained influence over the years with fellow workers that is necessary to be exercised in a crisis. This imperative adds support to the need for all employees to receive leadership training and development as healthcare organizations respond to the turbulent external environment.

Another area in which communication skills predominate is the articulation of the vision for the organization both inside the organization and to external stakeholders. According to Joshi and colleagues (2014), the vision and strategic plan of the healthcare organization cannot be effective in driving change unless it is communicated properly and continually. The leader's ability to communicate effectively the need for continuous quality improvement and cost reduction strategies for the entire healthcare organization has no substitute. These communications must represent the organization and must be understood by each employee, from physicians to custodians to registrars, if success is to be achieved.

This notion reflects the importance of developing charismatic power in formal and informal leaders alike. However, charismatic communications involve more than meeting with staff and promising them the leader has open availability for discussions. Charismatic leaders have the unique ability to gain the trust and cooperation of their followers by using their extraordinary communication skills. All employees must understand that gaining the ability to communicate charismatically takes time, effort, and dedication by the trainee. Clearly, a leader can learn quickly how to improve his communication skills. But above-average skills are limited in their impact unless the leader has the trust and belief of the employees that he is authentic. Some individuals are born with a charismatic communication ability; others can perform just as well by learning the skills and then being honest and trustworthy in all of their dealings with their fellow employees.

### Motivational and Employee Engagement Skills

Healthcare executives often tout the value of the organization's human capital, stating that staff are their most important resource. Remarkably, little attention is given to motivating employees. Fortunately, however, C-suite executives are beginning to realize the value of having motivated and engaged staff, especially during times of transformation.

The people who work in healthcare facilities are the direct link between the organization and its success or failure, and research has shown that appropriate motivation is one key to their achievement of high work performance, retention, and good organizational citizenship behavior. Elton and O'Riordan (2016) point out that organizational citizenship behavior is one area in the current (and necessary) metrics-driven world of performance improvement that is often overlooked in terms of organizational success. Staff who demonstrate good organizational citizenship speak positively about the organization when they connect with friends, family members, and acquaintances. This positive representation of the hospital or health system helps the organization attract new talent and maintain good community relationships. And it is through a motivated staff engaged in the improvement of care quality that organizations will remain viable through the next several years.

The responsibility for motivation and employee engagement in the process of work rests with the leaders of the organization and needs to be given top priority in any hierarchy of training needs. Healthcare employees must be motivated every day to find new ways to improve the quality of the services provided, a job that is never done in the ever-changing environment of healthcare delivery. Most of what we think we know about motivating individuals in the workplace is not only outdated but wrong, particularly for a team-based service delivery setting such as healthcare.

Pink (2009) argues that the workplace of scientific management guru Frederick Taylor has changed dramatically over the years, especially in the service sector, which comprises most of the current US economy. The work conducted in many service-sector jobs has become less routine, requiring creativity and offering increased satisfaction to the employee, a key intrinsic motivator (discussed in an earlier chapter). Pink (2009) further points out that employee satisfaction depends on meeting not only one's assigned goals but also the right goals, those holding the most intrinsic value for each employee.

The starting point for the healthcare organization leader in learning how to motivate and engage her employees in the workplace is to determine, on an individual basis, what motivates them. The common assumption is that when they started their work in the healthcare sector, these individuals were motivated by the prospect of delivering care-related services to people in need. That motivation may still be an important factor in the engagement of staff who have been working in healthcare for years, but the leader cannot count on that being the sole motivator for moving toward quality improvement and service excellence.

To gain skills in motivating and engaging employees in healthcare, the leader must appreciate the differences between extrinsic and intrinsic motivation. Compensation in the form of money and benefits (extrinsic motivators) is still an important performance incentive, but it is not as important as the feeling an employee experiences in creating value at work. The leader must communicate with her staff continuously to learn about—and remain in tune with—their essential motivators.

For example, according to Pink (2009), intrinsically motivated individuals who work in the service delivery sector usually do not require supervision to deliver superior service. A major dissatisfier for these employees is rooted in their perception that they do not have the organization's support or the necessary resources to deliver high-quality services. In this case, the leader needs to empower his employees to deliver the best care possible and be present to support them with the resources, emotional engagement, and training necessary to improve the quality of healthcare services offered.

## Culture-Building Skills

To be successful in meeting these and other challenges facing most healthcare organizations, cultural change, or in some cases cultural rebuilding, is required. The need for culture transformation is unquestioned, and it is the responsibility of the leader to effect such change. It is not an easy task, and the leader must understand the dangers associated with shifting an organizational culture that has been built and nurtured over a long period. Thus, culture-building skills are necessary for any leadership training and development program.

For example, the leader must learn how to communicate the importance of culture change to adequately manage the turbulent environment.

Empowering associates is another important aspect of culture change because the leader will need all the help he can get to hardwire the new culture. These elements and more should be components of a leadership development and training program considering, as noted in chapter 8, culture building is necessary for maximizing organizational performance.

### Trust-Building Skills

Perhaps underscoring all the skills noted in this section for inclusion in a leadership—and staff—development and training program is the presence of trust. A leader must gain the complete trust of both employees and consumers to successfully apply the other abilities. The importance of trust in organizational leadership is discussed at great length in chapter 7; here we focus on the training aspect of trust building.

Getting people to trust you is difficult when you are the one responsible for making them change the way they have conducted business for a long time, especially when they have been successful. Horsager (2009) points out that the opposite of trust is suspicion, which, if not overcome, has an enduring negative impact on employee motivation, the ability to work together as a team, and the quality of the final product or service.

Therefore, any leadership training and development program must devote time to helping the leader understand the value of trust and learn how to increase her level of trustworthiness. The starting point in the improvement of trust in the organization and its leadership is for the leader to gain a complete understanding of why healthcare employees have lost trust in the hospital or health system. Staff's reaction—and sometimes overreaction—to the changing healthcare environment has caused many formerly bureaucratic organizations to furlough employees, cut the benefits of remaining employees, and make other human resources mistakes as they attempt to deal with the unsettling shifts in the healthcare industry. Once the leader appreciates what the employees have been through over the past several years, she can understand why they are suspicious of any change. Training leaders to have this awareness is a cornerstone of healthcare leadership development and training programs.

### Intrapreneurship Skills

Empowering staff to be creative and innovative in healthcare services delivery can only occur in a decentralized organizational structure with workers who are encouraged to resolve issues using proven problem-solving approaches. Many healthcare observers believe the best way to improve quality and reduce the cost of healthcare delivery is by tapping the skills found in an entrepreneur working with a start-up company, as discussed in an earlier chapter in terms of dual organizational structure. This realization has led a number of healthcare organizations to consider adopting a culture of intrapreneurship.

Intrapreneurship is seen in an individual or a group of individuals who behave like entrepreneurs but work for a larger organization than the typical start-up company. This concept needs to receive appropriate attention from healthcare organizations as they attempt to reform and reengineer their organizations. Part of that effort should be to develop leaders and staff in skills related to intrapreneurship.

Samit (2015) describes an intrapreneur as an individual who has been empowered by his workplace to combine the innovative freedom of a start-up company with the resources available from inside a large organization. The intrapreneur thus is afforded the ability to focus on creativity and innovation, forcing radical change on an organization. This application of a dual organizational structure has been adopted successfully in many nonhealthcare organizations.

Intrapreneurship allows for the best of both worlds: enjoying the thrill of entrepreneurship with little fear of personal risk. Creating something new while facing numerous operational challenges is rewarding for staff because the process often results in the successful utilization of innovation. It also offers the employee the opportunity to experience the flow concept described by Csikszentmihaly (2009). Obviously, the opportunity to practice intrapreneurship could be an intrinsic motivator for many employees.

Tapping intrapreneurship skills also allows an organization to disrupt itself before an outside hostile competitor causes the disruption. Herbold (2007) notes the contention of many observers that if camera and film company Kodak had used this strategy many years ago, it would have been in a position to take advantage of the digital film innovation and not gone bankrupt. The problem faced by Kodak is similar to the threats hospitals encounter today, with many of their services being threatened by outside competitors looking to profit from their disruption.

The universal reason given for not practicing intrapreneurship is fear of failure. The healthcare leader is responsible to not only gain a solid understanding of intrapreneurship but also encourage staff to practice it continually. The leader's skills in and understanding of intrapreneurship are the key to implementing it successfully in a culture; only he can provide the ideal environment that supports this creativity for employees who wish to think outside the normal parameters of operations to solve pressing challenges.

## Evaluation of Leadership Development Programs

One of the most important components of the leadership training and development program is a well-developed evaluation of the success or failure of the new program. Evaluating the outcomes of a training program is typically not a popular task for any program manager, but it provides invaluable information for improving the leadership training process.

The evaluation process must be included in the framework of the development program at the outset, at the same time the program objectives are developed. If planned and executed properly, the evaluation offers support for continuing the program by attracting additional resources once its advantages are known, and it lends insight on strategies to improve it. The evaluation process allows the organization to measure training outcomes and helps its developers identify needed revisions to the program.

A simple approach to evaluating a leadership training and development program is to employ a systems model, including input, throughput, and output, to test the effectiveness of different training methods. Exhibit 10.3 shows the systems approach to evaluating the conflict management component of a leadership training module.

In this exhibit, the conflict management training program is the input. It must include the objectives to be achieved by offering the program for prospective leaders of the healthcare organization. Once the objectives are outlined, a specific educational program is developed and offered to the chosen employees as the throughput phase of the program. The output of this conflict management training module should be improved conflict management skills for the training program participants. Because the objectives of this program are built into its input phase, measuring whether they are achieved in the output phase of this program is straightforward. If improvement in the particular skills is not proven in the evaluation, the program requires further development to make sure the skills are aquired through the program.

Donald Kirkpatrick is thought to have developed, in 1959, one of the best models for measuring the results of learning programs (Bock 2015). This model includes four levels along which organizations can determine the success of a training program:

- Reaction
- Learning
- Behavior
- Results

According to Bock (2015), the first level of Kirkpatrick's model measures the extent to which learners react to a training program. It gauges whether the learners are engaged in the training process and think it is worthwhile for their leadership development. Although perhaps not the most important aspect of a leadership development program, the students' satisfaction with the content of the program and the instructor who conducted it is essential for the program's success.

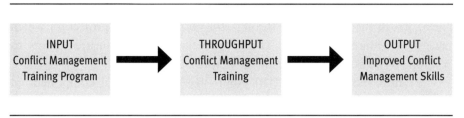

**EXHIBIT 10.3**
Conflict
Management
Training Module

The second phase of Kirkpatrick's model relates to the actual learning that takes place during the program. This stage represents the reason for the training effort because its essential aim is to change knowledge or attitudes of trainees.

The third level assesses the behavior change that should occur as a result of this educational endeavor. The new behaviors should allow leaders to become active throughout the organization despite their lack of position power. They have now gained empowerment to improve the value of their services as they attempt to meet all of the needs of their patients on a daily basis.

The final phase of Kirkpatrick's training program evaluation model determines the results achieved by attendees. This phase captures the improvements to leadership skill seen in participants as an outcome of the training.

## Creating a Leadership Development Program: How to Begin

For strong leadership to be a factor in effecting change and leading for service excellence, organizations must analyze their structure to determine whether it is bureaucratic, decentralized, or another type. This determination spurs many healthcare organizations operating as a bureaucracy run by healthcare managers to reorganize to be more decentralized, requiring leadership rather than management.

Whether these future leaders come from the ranks of healthcare management or move into healthcare delivery from another discipline, all require leadership development and training to prepare their organizations for the future manifestations of healthcare delivery.

Bennis (2009) cautions that leaders are never made by taking a corporate training program or even college courses in business administration. The real education that makes a leader is the experience he gains by leading others toward the achievement of goals. Therefore, establishing an organizational commitment to develop leaders, providing them with opportunities to learn through experience and mistakes, makes more sense than requiring formal training alone.

**Internship**
On-the-job training that may be offered by a college for academic credit.

Prospective leaders also may benefit from an **internship** experience during which they lead people through the completion of a project for which success or failure is assessed. These opportunities allow future leaders to develop all the skills discussed in this chapter.

White and Griffith (2016) emphasize that a critical component of an excellent healthcare organization is its investment in leadership development and training programs for current and future leaders as well as staff. Furthermore, they note that such programs must be viewed as long-term investments. They cost money in the short term but should lead to improved quality of healthcare services and reduced costs for the organization in the future. One consequence, of course, is that those who receive the benefits of training and development programs may leave the organization, taking the organization's investment with them. While this is a valid consideration in planning a leadership development and training program, it may be short-sighted and potentially devalues the very employees touted as the organization's most important resource.

## Summary

For healthcare leaders to improve the quality of healthcare services while reducing the costs of delivering those services, they must acquire and master many new skills. These include team leadership, communication, motivation and employee engagement, and intrapreneurship as well as culture building and trust building.

Particularly important among these is the ability to communicate with employees and customers. Communication skills are often taken for granted by superiors when an individual moves into a leadership position. This oversight can hinder the leader's development if she is in fact a poor communicator.

Another key skill area for healthcare leaders to develop is motivating and engaging employees in the process of work. Healthcare employees need to be motivated every day to find new ways to improve the quality of the services delivered. The need for improvement never ends in the ever-changing environment of the healthcare industry.

## Discussion Questions

1. Why is leadership training so important for healthcare organizations?
2. Explain the needs assessment process as it relates to leadership training and development.

3. Explain the evaluation process of leadership training and development programs.

4. Name and explain some of the most important skills to be gained in a leadership training and development program.

# References

Bandura, A. 1976. *Social Learning Theory.* New York: Pearson.

Becker, E., and J. Wortman. 2009. *Mastering Communications at Work: How to Lead, Manage, and Influence.* New York: McGraw-Hill.

Bennis, W. 2009. *On Becoming a Leader.* New York: Basic.

Bock, L. 2015. *Work Rules! Insights from Inside Google That Will Transform How You Live and Lead.* New York: Twelve.

Bolden, R., B. Hawkins, J. Gosling, and S. Taylor. 2011. *Exploring Leadership: Individual, Organizational & Societal Perspectives.* New York: Oxford University Press.

Csikszentmihaly, M. 2009. *Flow.* New York: Harper Collins.

Elsner, R., and B. Farrands. 2006. *Leadership Transitions: How Business Leaders Take Charge in New Roles.* Philadelphia, PA: Kogan Page.

Elton, J., and A. O'Riordan. 2016. *Healthcare Disrupted: Next Generation Business Models and Strategies.* Hoboken, NJ: Wiley.

Herbold, R. J. 2007. *Seduced by Success: How the Best Companies Survive the 9 Traps of Winning.* New York: McGraw-Hill.

Hill, L. A., G. Brandeau, E. Truelove, and K. Lineback. 2014. *Collective Genius: The Art and Practice of Leading Innovation.* Boston: Harvard Business Review Press.

Horsager, D. 2009. *The Trust Edge: How Top Leaders Gain Faster Results, Deeper Relationships, and a Stronger Bottom Line.* New York: Free Press.

Joshi, M. S., E. R. Ransom, D. B. Nash, and S. B. Ransom. 2014. *The Healthcare Quality Book: Vision, Strategy, and Tools.* Chicago: Health Administration Press.

Karlgaard, R., and M. S. Malone. 2015. *Team Genius: The New Science of High-Performing Organizations.* New York: Harper Business.

Nahavandi, A. 2015. *The Art and Science of Leadership,* 7th ed. New York: Pearson.

Pink, D. H. 2009. *Drive: The Surprising Truth About What Motivates Us.* New York: Riverhead.

Samit, J. 2015. *Disrupt You: Master Personal Transformation, Seize Opportunity, and Thrive in the Era of Endless Innovation.* New York: Flatiron.

White, K. R., and J. R. Griffith. 2016. *The Well-Managed Healthcare Organization,* 8th ed. Chicago: Health Administration Press.

# PHYSICIAN CEOS AS LEADERS OF HEALTHCARE ORGANIZATIONS

Francis G. Belardi

> A true leader has the confidence to stand alone, the courage to make tough decisions, and the compassion to listen to the needs of others. He does not set out to be a leader, but becomes one by the equality of his actions and the integrity of his intent.
>
> —Gen. Douglas MacArthur

## Learning Objectives

After completing this chapter, readers should be able to

- describe the need for physician leadership training,
- discuss the role of the patient-centered medical home in the US healthcare system,
- explain the different models of physician leadership in healthcare delivery, and
- summarize the role of the integrated healthcare system in healthcare delivery.

## Key Terms and Concepts

- Administrative model
- American Association for Physician Leadership
- Dyad model
- Emotional intelligence
- Hybrid educational model
- Institute for Healthcare Improvement (IHI)
- Integrated healthcare system
- Managed care
- Patient-centered medical home (PCMH)

## Introduction

Never before in the history of modern medicine in the United States has physician leadership been pivotal to the success of the healthcare delivery system. It is today.

With the delivery of modern healthcare, **managed care** has emerged from a fragmented system, capitated payments have become the cornerstone of reimbursement, and the operational paradigm has shifted to value-based reimbursement. Financial penalties are already in place for those healthcare organizations that do not make the shift to value-based care, and these penalties will no doubt increase with time and because of additional financial constraints expected to be imposed by government payers such as Medicare and Medicaid. During the past five years, the Affordable Care Act (ACA) has been enacted in phases, and this legislation has added covered lives to the health insurance rolls—a clear benefit for millions of US residents but an additional burden on an already stressed healthcare system.

With the rapidly changing healthcare landscape, US physicians can no longer be content to provide healthcare alone, deferring operational decisions to administrators, many of whom are nonphysicians. The call for physicians now is to actively participate in shaping the new delivery system to meet the Triple Aim of the **Institute of Healthcare Improvement (IHI)**: improving quality and patient satisfaction, improving the health of populations, and reducing the cost of healthcare delivery (Berwick, Nolan, and Whittington 2008; IHI 2016).

For physicians to effect change and achieve the Triple Aim, they must embrace new models of care, such as the **patient-centered medical home (PCMH)**. Additionally, a significant number of physicians must transform their roles from independent providers to leaders in the new healthcare landscape. Physician leaders of the past were found in roles such as chair of a clinical department or chief of the medical staff. Current and future leaders must assume broader responsibilities, such as those assigned to a chief quality officer, chief of medical informatics, or patient safety officer, residing in the hospital or health system C-suite instead of the medical staff center. This transformation requires significant additional training beyond medical school so that physicians learn the business of medicine.

**Managed care**
Techniques adopted by third-party payers to reduce the cost and improve the quality of healthcare.

**Institute for Healthcare Improvement (IHI)**
Organization dedicated to improving healthcare services worldwide.

**Patient-centered medical home (PCMH)**
A care delivery model in which healthcare is provided and coordinated through a primary care doctor.

## History of Physician Leadership

Physicians have begun realizing the mandate for assuming additional roles in shaping the future of the US healthcare system. Historically, US physicians were self-employed entrepreneurs, and their primary function was to provide direct patient care in the office and hospital settings. Physicians did not traditionally assume administrative or leadership roles until later in their careers and often accepted a leadership role as a bridge from clinical practice to retirement. Few of the past leaders ever had any formal leadership training.

In that historical paradigm, the hospital was the only arena that required some form of physician leadership to develop and manage hospital clinical services. Several leadership roles emerged, such as chairs of clinical departments supported by clinical section chiefs. For example, a chair of medicine would be appointed to manage the adult medical services subspecialties of cardiology, endocrinology, critical care, nephrology, and the like. Section chiefs, with specific knowledge in their disciplines, were appointed to lead their subspecialties.

All these appointments were made on the basis of the collective perception of the appointed leaders' clinical excellence. Leaders were not chosen for their business acumen or experience. This model became the first type of dyad approach to healthcare leadership: Nonphysicians managed the business operations of hospitals in conjunction with physicians who managed the clinical spectrum of healthcare delivery and services. The roles and responsibilities were separate and distinct but complementary. The **dyad model** has persisted for many decades because medical training did not include education in business or management and few physicians pursued advanced degrees in medical management or business administration.

The landmark article by Stoller (2008) on the development of physician leaders reviews the history of physician leadership development in the United States dating back to 1950 and outlines the competencies required for physician leaders and the types of educational programs available to train physician leaders.

More recently, a number of health systems have merged into **integrated healthcare systems**. As they have formed, some have been led by physicians who received leadership training. These physician leaders recognized the need for development of other physician leaders necessary to advance the healthcare organization and to provide bench strength for succession planning.

Increasing numbers of physicians enrolled in physician leadership certificate programs or sought master's degrees in business administration, medical management, or health administration at established universities. Some integrated healthcare systems instituted their own leadership programs, and others funded the additional training in master's-level education courses or similar programs.

In 2014, about 5 percent of healthcare systems were led by physician CEOs, and the top five healthcare systems in the United States were under the leadership of a physician CEO (Angood and Birk 2014). This statistic

**Dyad model**
An approach to leadership in which the physician leader and administrative leader work together in distinct but complementary roles.

**Integrated healthcare system**
An organizational arrangement that focuses on the coordination of patient care.

offers a sharp contrast to the physician leadership void in healthcare organizations of the prior 25 years. The changing healthcare insurance landscape and governmental initiatives have caught the attention of physicians, encouraging or compelling some to pursue higher-level administrative leadership roles.

## Physician Leader Competencies

The desire to change medicine for the better is only the beginning of the journey to physician leadership. In past years, the requirements for physician leadership were only clinical excellence and a desire to lead. Clinical excellence remains an important attribute for physician leaders because rank-and-file practitioners seem to trust clinical leaders more than those with an administrative background. The physician CEOs at respected US medical institutions (e.g., Johns Hopkins Medicine, Mayo Clinic, Cleveland Clinic) have had distinguished medical careers marked by recognized clinical credibility.

Clinical credibility and excellence combined with leadership desire, however, is insufficient for physicians to be effective leaders today. Competencies for effective physician leadership fall into the following categories: knowledge of the past and evolving healthcare system; vision; trust and respect; ability to collaborate and delegate, including effective communication skills; and **emotional intelligence** (Farrell and Robbins 1993; McKenna Gartland, and Pugno 2004).

**Emotional intelligence**
The ability to have a keen awareness of others' emotions and to effectively express and control one's own emotions when dealing with others.

### *Healthcare System Knowledge*

Knowledge of healthcare systems, past, present, and evolving, is a primary competency for physician leadership. Just as one must achieve competence in one's medical discipline, a physician leader must achieve a complete understanding of business and learn the language used in business matters. This level of understanding includes healthcare system finance and how to achieve margins to invest in system growth. An in-depth knowledge of healthcare law beyond professional liability also is mandatory. Information technology knowledge beyond billing systems and electronic health records is required, and Lean and Six Sigma must be learned in the context of developing an efficient delivery system.

The health system knowledge competency must be gained in a structured academic program, preferably one that confers a recognized credential such as a certificate in physician leadership or an accredited master's degree program.

### *Vision*

The physician leader must be a visionary. Strategic planning and execution are the outcomes of vision and as such are critical leadership skills. The leader must develop an expectation of—a vision for—his healthcare system and how that expectation dovetails with the bigger picture of national healthcare. The vision clearly must be realistic, be supported by data, be financially viable, and produce high-quality outcomes.

## Trust and Respect

Trust and respect are imperative to leadership effectiveness and success in all types of leadership, including physician leadership. Subordinates follow those they trust. An effective leadership chain recognizes trust in the physician leader and inspires and models that trust in those that govern. A single breach of trust is enough to seriously impair leadership effectiveness. Healthcare system leaders do not differ from their counterparts in the nonmedical world with regard to the consequences for breach of trust. The Enron Corporation scandal of 2001 is one of many examples that captures the effects of breach-of-trust consequences for investors, employees, corporations, and their leaders. In addition to the bankruptcy and dissolution of the corporation, CEO Kenneth Lay was indicted for multiple counts of security fraud and faced trial and imprisonment. Shareholders filed multiple lawsuits, and employees lost their jobs (Frontain 2017). Medical corporations and their leaders would not be immune from similar consequences.

## Collaboration, Delegation, and Communication

Physician leaders must be collaborators and delegators. No leader can possibly manage the myriad day-to-day functions of an organization; its effectiveness depends on multilevel collaboration and delegation while holding the chain of leadership accountable.

To do so, verbal, written, and nonverbal communication skills are essential. Furthermore, the physician leader must learn which mode of communication is appropriate in a given circumstance. Those who are led want to see their leaders, hear their vision captured in words, and be motivated to succeed.

## Emotional Intelligence

Finally, to be effective, the physician leader must be emotionally intelligent. Emotional intelligence is the ability to be aware of one's emotions and to regulate and manage those emotions effectively in dealing with the emotions of others. Physicians are trained in the medical model to react. Physician leaders must learn to respond. Consider the physician-practitioner managing a cardiac arrest. She must react immediately and follow protocol in an emotionally charged situation. The physician leader must respond to critical situations, but she usually has time to pause and reflect on the situation before a decision is required. Emotional intelligence in all physician leadership situations is characterized by calm and reassurance. Followers who have trust in their physician leader are guided in part by the emotional intelligence she displays, enabling the team to respond to and solve problems effectively.

The physician leader who possesses all the competencies but lacks emotional intelligence likely will not succeed. Because leadership is a fluid state, the physician leader constantly must be aware of his image and regulate his behavior to adjust to variable situations. The physician leader must understand that his decisions may not always lead the organization down the correct path, and the emotionally intelligent leader must (1) have the courage to admit to his team that a previous decision proved ineffective and (2) be willing to move in a different direction. Such humility is a desirable leadership trait; it is perceived positively by the team and strengthens the physician leader's image.

## The Cascading of Physician Leadership Education and Training

In the medical model of leadership, physicians are accustomed to giving orders and expecting an immediate response and often immediate results. The paradigm shift to the **administrative model** requires a different mindset. Physicians who want to lead must learn that change in organizations is almost always incremental and rarely transformational. Physician leaders must learn to deal with ambiguity frequently and not rely on the medical model of transformational results.

**Administrative model**
An approach to leadership that relies on a nonmedical healthcare manager for efficiency.

The transformation from clinician to leader involves a long process of new learning and experiences. Physicians in medical practice require *patients* for professional success, while physicians in leadership roles must model *patience*.

Much as the desire to be a physician practitioner involves a commitment to education averaging 12 years, the wish to become a physician leader is the beginning of a lengthy journey. Physician executives undergo formal education as well as training and experience through progressive leadership roles throughout their careers. That cascading of leadership training for physician leaders to reach the top of the leadership hierarchy may take an additional 10 to 12 years.

A common leadership myth is that leaders are born and not made. We suggest that the reality is quite the opposite. Certainly, particular personality traits are recognized attributes in most leaders, such as good social skills, good communication skills, and trust building. However, many of the critical leadership skills must be learned, similar to learning the critical skills of medical practice.

An individual who desires to be a physician engages in a defined process that includes premedical education, medical school education, residency, fellowship, and more depending on the type of practice. Each step adds medical knowledge, clinical experience, and increasing responsibility for the well-being of patients. Likewise, a physician whose goal is to become a hospital or healthcare system CEO must traverse a leadership cascade built on administrative and operational system knowledge, leadership experience, and increasing responsibility for the efficient operations of individuals, teams, and organizational entities. Such cascading begins with the physician's role as a practitioner leading a small team managing a specific patient population. The physician then may become part of larger organizational teams, such as a clinical quality committee, pharmacy and therapeutics committee, medical records committee, ethics committee, or a similar group. As the physician acquires system knowledge and earns the trust and respect of others, she may assume more responsible roles as specialty division chief, where her scope of influence is further increased. Eventually, she may take on a department chair or service line director role, which increases her organizational visibility, knowledge, and accountability.

Successive appointments and roles may include election to boards, promotion to medical directorships, or elevation to head of a group of service lines, with the ultimate achievement being a move to healthcare system president/CEO for some.

Simultaneously, physician leaders must achieve specific leadership knowledge through an established, credible certifying agency. One such national organization is the **American Association for Physician Leadership** (formerly the American College of Physician Executives), among the first organizations to recognize the need for physician leadership education and provide an educational framework to achieve the necessary leadership skills. The American College of Healthcare Executives, the premier organization for healthcare executives, also provides physicians with educational and networking opportunities that are critical to building leadership skills.

In addition, many integrated healthcare systems now provide leadership education for physicians through internal certificate programs that aim to provide the leadership skills necessary for the early phases of physician leadership, starting with section chief–level capabilities and moving into department chair roles. Finally, master's degree programs can provide enhanced skills for intermediate levels of physician leadership, such as medical directorships, executives of medical groups, CEOs of small hospitals, and so on. Master's programs are typically offered by colleges and universities, but an emerging physician leadership training model features the development of skills at the academic medical center or in a collaborative relationship between the university and healthcare system.

**American Association for Physician Leadership**
A professional association that focuses on training and supporting physicians to hold hospital and health system leadership positions.

**Hybrid educational model**
Combines a traditional face-to-face class with outside classroom experiences.

Such **hybrid educational models,** whereby much of the education is provided via the Internet or teleclasses, with only a portion of the time being spent at the academic institution, are appealing to many physicians who pursue leadership training for a variety of personal and professional reasons. Numerous competing priorities in physicians' lives have historically prevented physicians from pursuing and completing leadership training. This type of hybrid educational program permits the physician to obtain the necessary education without frequent travel to an academic center while helping to ensure continuity of the physicians' practice, maintenance of clinical productivity, provision for appropriate work–life balance, and reduction in costs associated with travel and in-class tuition.

Healthcare organizations that employ physician practitioners embrace the hybrid model as well. They can contain costs to educate clinicians who desire the advanced training, reduce lost productivity time, and retain those physicians, as the funding of leadership education by the organization is usually tied to a contractual agreement for years of future services. This model can represent a win–win for the healthcare system and the individual physician.

Once the physician leader has obtained the academic skills and progressive experience through the leadership cascade, he should participate in a talent management program that provides mentoring and leadership effectiveness evaluation. Talent management is a human resources initiative with a goal to create high-performing, engaged employees throughout an organization. Talent management is not unique to medicine and has been used in nonmedical organizations for some time to evaluate and mentor leadership effectiveness. Many healthcare organizations now recognize the value of talent management programs for physician leaders (Brightman 2007; Satiani et al. 2014).

One valuable aspect of talent management programs is that they offer a process for measuring leadership effectiveness on an annual basis. In general, 360-degree evaluation systems use input from individuals in corporations who have leadership-related interactions with the evaluee. Input is solicited from those to whom the leader reports, those who report to the leader, and the leader's peers, creating a panoramic view of the leader's performance. The assessment used is a variant of the 360-degree evaluation system as part of a validated, commercially available talent management software program and includes both physicians and nonphysicians in the evaluator mix (Olivo 2014). The reports from the assessment are used both to improve the performance of physician leaders who lag in their progress and to move average or high performers further along on their journey to leadership excellence.

To supplement the assessment process, particularly for underperforming physician leaders, another key component of talent management is coaching on a regular basis. Coaching frequency depends on the results of the physician leader profile. The profile is generated from the input obtained via the assessment tool, which measures the physician leader on the competencies previously mentioned and defined. For example, a leader who excels in most aspects of leadership may be coached every three months, whereas a leader who has failed to grasp the fundamental competencies of leadership may need weekly or biweekly coaching. Coaching can include one-on-one discussions with the coach, completion of online leadership training modules, participation in advanced leadership training seminars, and similar activities.

Physician leaders should not expect to achieve success in leadership roles without ongoing evaluation and measurement of their leadership effectiveness. Talent management assessment should not be a foreign concept to physician leaders, as physicians by now are accustomed to a similar process in their clinical roles. Maintenance of certification (MOC) in clinical practice has been required for the past decade by many medical specialties to retain their board certification. In the recent past, a physician who achieved board certification in her medical specialty would be certified for life. With the rapid expansion of medical knowledge and increased complexity of medicine, the national medical specialty hierarchy (including the leadership of national medical specialty organizations, e.g., American Board of Medical Specialties, and other medical and surgical specialty boards, e.g., American Board of Internal Medicine, American Board of Surgery) instituted MOC. Certification maintenance requires periodic cognitive examinations to maintain board certification, usually every ten years, as well as completion of annual educational modules on specialty-specific topics and practice improvement modules based on actual patient care in the respective physician's practice. The talent management process is expected to emerge as the "leadership MOC" for current and future physician leaders.

Often the talent management approach fails to improve an individual physician's leadership effectiveness and the organization must make the critical decision to replace the ineffective leader. Although the talent management process cannot guarantee that all aspiring physician leaders succeed, it is invaluable in helping hospital and healthcare system leaders identify physicians who are progressing well and those who are failing, and working with them accordingly.

## Measuring Success of Physician Leaders

In the current healthcare system, CEOs tend to be measured by a single metric: financial margin, and the magnitude of that margin. Healthcare margins are considerably lower than those of nonhealthcare industries. The average healthcare system margin of 2 percent is considered a successful achievement, and many healthcare systems do not even gain a positive margin consistently.

Financial margins historically have been driven by service volume. In the newer models of care, the focus is shifting from volume-driven reimbursement to value-based reimbursement. In past systems, effort was rewarded financially, but in the new systems, outcomes are entered into the payment equation. As such, healthcare systems with low patient satisfaction scores, higher-than-average patient mortality rates, and poor clinical outcomes will be financially penalized regardless of volume.

The Centers for Medicare & Medicaid Services (CMS) has been the leader in developing quantifiable metrics to assess healthcare system performance during the past several years. Quality assessment historically had been limited to hospital performance until recently. In 2017, new programs for quality payments to physicians and physician extenders will become the law. The global legislation known as MACRA (the Medicare Access and CHIP Reauthorization Act) includes the Merit-Based Incentive Payment System and Alternative Payment Models. The metrics required by MACRA are numerous and available for public view on the CMS website (www.cms.gov).

Physician leaders can have a tremendous impact on clinical outcomes. Physicians have the knowledge, training, and experience to alter the course of disease outcomes, such as by reducing hospital infection rates, improving all-cause mortality rates, and reducing or eliminating never events involving hospitalized patients that frequently result in unnecessary complications with prolonged hospital stays or, even worse, patient deaths.

Physician leaders must harness all this knowledge by developing and monitoring accurate and reliable clinical outcome dashboards and scorecards for individual practitioners and for the healthcare system in the aggregate. The data from these dashboards is used to improve the health of populations, especially in those with chronic diseases such as diabetes mellitus and congestive heart failure. Poor control of diabetes and heart failure leads to repetitive hospital admissions and high financial cost for the healthcare system in general as well as increased costs to third-party payers. Insurers have begun refusing to pay for hospital readmissions within 30 days postdischarge, and that trend will only increase.

In addition to clinical accountability, physician leaders must be financially accountable to ensure the fiscal viability of the healthcare system. This role requires understanding and applying appropriate clinical and nonclinical staffing ratios, continuous upgrading of technology to enhance and support clinical service lines, appropriate contracting with third-party payers, and other complex administrative activities. Furthermore, the expenses attached to these initiatives need to be balanced with healthcare system profitability. The saying "No margin, no mission" captures the essence of financial viability.

Physicians are the drivers of any healthcare system, and physician leaders must recruit and retain competent physician talent. Fulfilling this responsibility requires a fair and transparent compensation model. Medical group annual turnover rate is one solid metric by which to determine physician alignment and success. Physician and physician extender turnover rates of less than 7 percent in group practice models associated with integrated healthcare system models are ideal. Turnover rate is another metric indicating the overall effectiveness of physician leadership. Physicians and extenders always tend to look for "greener pastures," but the assumption is that lower turnover rates imply a high correlation with physician and extender happiness with their current healthcare system and its leadership.

Although compensation is a key consideration in recruitment and retention of physicians, it is not the only one. Other factors include workload expectations, work–life balance, availability of leadership opportunities, and availability of employment opportunities in the community for spouses. Each healthcare system has unique challenges depending on geography and local economies, and physician leaders must understand their implications.

Physician leaders must also ensure that their healthcare system supports the necessary IT infrastructure to provide all appropriate clinical and financial data necessary to conduct assessments of performance and initiate adjustments to processes. Most physicians understand clinical IT software and its applications, and certainly this understanding is invaluable in their leadership duties as well. A comprehensive patient care IT infrastructure includes the electronic health record (EHR); scheduling and billing software; computerized provider order entry; and radiological imaging and laboratory reporting, retrieval, and archival software. These IT domains touch nearly every patient in the healthcare system, and a robust EHR does far more. The ideal EHR contains a registry function to assess quality in population management, evidence-based medical reference materials, patient education materials, clinical decision support tools, and many other components.

Where most physician leaders need new IT skills is on the business side of care delivery. Many software applications are available to provide business intelligence (BI) needed to interpret key nonclinical system performance data, such as key performance indicators, supply cost data, regulatory compliance data, risk management data, revenue cycle data, and patient flow information, to name just a few BI areas.

*Data* and *outcomes* are two current buzzwords relevant to modern healthcare leaders. Physicians are trained in clinical decision making on the basis of data, and this is a strength many physician leaders bring to leadership.

# Debates Surrounding Physician Leaders

### Physician CEOs Versus Nonphysician CEOs

Much debate has been waged regarding hospital and health system performance under physician CEOs versus nonphysician CEOs. Historically, nonphysician CEOs have dominated healthcare system leadership, and currently, only 5 percent of healthcare systems are led by physician CEOs.

One hypothesis posits that healthcare system performance could improve under physician CEOs as the physician CEO adds the "clinical lens" perspective through which to view operational and strategic governance (Goodall 2011). Little conclusive research exists to validate this perspective, however. It will take a few generations of physicians with leadership aspirations and training to change the balance of healthcare system leadership. In the interim, a solution that balances the skill sets of physician CEOs and nonphysician CEOs must be created.

Intuitive reasoning suggests that physician CEOs and nonphysician CEOs bring complementary influence and skills to the executive suite. Nonphysician CEOs traditionally excel at operating under the business model while physician CEOs excel under a clinical integration model. Rather than an either–or choice for healthcare system leadership, an expanded dyad model has been suggested as a reasonable solution (Zismer and Brueggeman 2010). Ideally, the combined leadership skill set leverages skills from across the spectrum of medical leadership.

The question has been raised whether a co-CEO dyad structure equates to a no-CEO result. Not necessarily, in the author's experience. However, the co-CEO dyad must be founded on reciprocal trust and mutual accountability to achieve positive results in the value-based reimbursement model.

### Physicians as Leaders: Will the New Paradigm Work?

Physicians serving as leaders of healthcare systems represent a new paradigm for the US healthcare system. Hospitals and other healthcare organizations have been managed and sustained for decades by nonphysician CEOs and director boards composed of nonphysician business executives. Why then should the business of medicine rest with physician leaders who may be seen as usurping their executive roles for personal gain (Blendon, Benson, and Hero 2014)? Despite public opinion regarding distrust of physicians (Gallup 2016), many physicians have impeccable professionalism and altruism and assume leadership roles as a means to change medicine for the better. Most physicians embrace high quality, compassion, and patient satisfaction in their daily work. Increasing numbers of physicians are willing to accept leadership roles and invest personal time to obtain the requisite training for leadership while continuing to provide direct patient care. For many physician leaders, coexistent part-time clinical practice is mandatory.

Rather than look at an either–or choice for executive healthcare leadership, the executive dyad model of healthcare leadership again offers a reasonable alternative. In the executive dyad model the strengths of physician leadership and nonphysician leadership are combined, offering a harmonizing skill set to healthcare leadership. In the dyad-led healthcare system, collaboration, shared decision making, and unified stance are mandatory.

There have been few executive dyad-led healthcare systems nationally to judge overall success or failure of this leadership style; however, the model is clearly worth exploring as healthcare system complexity increases.

## Future Physician Leadership Challenges

The next 10 to 15 years will be a critical time for the assessment of physicians as leaders. Current and emerging issues will challenge physician leaders, and the results of those tests will either ensure the physician executives' place at the leadership table or discredit their aspirations to lead healthcare systems.

A complete listing and discussion of all the issues facing future physician leaders—and healthcare leadership in general—is beyond the scope of this chapter. The following issues will appear on the agendas of physician leaders who govern large, integrated medical groups and healthcare systems:

- New healthcare legislation and possible repeal of or amendment to the ACA
- New models of care beyond accountable care organizations (ACOs) and the PCMH
- Emerging role of physician extenders—nurse practitioners, physician assistants, midwives, and so on
- Advanced IT and healthcare IT interoperability
- Alignment issues with employed physicians
- Physician recruitment and retention in group and integrated models
- Projected shortage of physicians
- Aging population and end-of-life care
- Integration of behavioral sciences in healthcare reform
- Reimbursement and bundled payments
- Unionization of physicians
- Telemedicine
- Medical consumerism and medical tourism
- Disruptive technologies and disruptive innovation

- Quality and patient safety
- Physician burnout

### Federal Healthcare Legislation

The ACA has been a transformational piece of healthcare legislation, changing the medical practice and insurance landscapes much like Medicare transformed eldercare in the 1960s. Having survived congressional repeal efforts and court proceedings to declare the 2010 healthcare reform legislation unconstitutional, the ACA faces future challenges as the executive and congressional branches of the federal government shift in 2017. Physician leaders need to participate in these legislative discussions, as physician input is critical to shape the future of national healthcare whether the US healthcare system becomes a single-payer system or remains in its present form.

### New Models of Care Delivery

New models of care for population management may emerge beyond ACOs and PCMHs. The PCMH concept has been generally accepted by the primary care community for its team-based approach to population management. ACO growth has been slower to achieve acceptance in the healthcare environment. As more healthcare systems merge into larger and larger entities over the next decade, newer models of care will probably emerge.

### Physician Extenders

Physician extenders have already become a disruptive force to traditional physician practice. Originally envisioned to support physician practices, physician extenders are increasingly seeking independent privileges and enhanced professional fees for the professional services they render. Physician leaders must develop a collaborative strategy to define the roles of these practitioners in the complex healthcare system of the future in a way that balances the needs of patients and the livelihoods of physicians with physician extenders' expectations of remuneration and professional satisfaction.

### Advanced Information Technology and Interoperability

The US healthcare system of the future will require unprecedented volumes of data to support clinical quality assessment. The federal government has taken the lead in this arena with programs such as the Physician Quality Reporting System, which assesses the quality of medical care delivered to Medicare beneficiaries. Physicians often question the data reported in this type of system. The literature suggests that doctors are often skeptical of the validity of data collection, have difficulty interpreting complex data reporting systems, and have concerns about the potential negative effects of public data reporting on their professional reputation (Barr et al. 2008). Physician leaders have the opportunity to influence the construction of validated quality reporting systems to drive positive changes in patient population management. To do so, physician leaders will require advanced training in data analytics to analyze and incorporate clinical data into population health management practices.

Health information technology interoperability remains a challenge for future physician leaders. The ability of EHRs to communicate with each other, exchange data, and use those data to achieve improved patient outcomes would promote coordination of care from the primary care office to the tertiary care institution. Pooled data across EHR systems could also significantly enhance practice-based clinical research, which would improve quality and outcomes. Physician leaders will need to develop strategies with EHR vendors and the government to break down the barriers to data exchange while maintaining patient confidentiality.

### Employed Physicians

More and more physicians and physician extenders are seeking employment in group practices or integrated healthcare systems. Often, however, the desires for employment do not coincide with group ideology or mission and vision alignment. In seeking employment arrangements, medical providers desire job and financial security, especially during times of change and uncertainty, such as a guaranteed salary, benefits, and protected vacation time. They may promise loyalty and commitment to groups in return for the benefits. Often these providers are short-term players and transition to other positions where the "grass looks greener." This movement affects turnover rate and medical group stability, with the additional concern of recruitment cost for replacement.

### Physician Recruitment and Retention

Some physicians have ideological and philosophical conflicts with the concept and practice of being employed and may become disruptive when their autonomous, private-practice style is threatened. Physician leaders must focus on selecting the appropriate practitioners for the health system medical practice by embedding sophisticated behavioral interviewing techniques in the recruitment process. In addition, they should develop a balanced retention program to preserve the best talent and reduce turnover. Physician leaders will need to develop attractive compensation models and promote acceptable and attractive work–life balance options as well.

### Physician Shortages

Several governmental agencies and medical associations such as the American Association of Medical Colleges and the American Medical Association have predicted a shortage of approximately 90,000 to 130,000 US-trained physicians by 2030, and a third of this deficit (roughly 40,000 physicians) is estimated to be seen in the primary care specialties. As the nation's population has increased and the demand for healthcare services has grown due to passage of the ACA, medical school output has not increased appreciably to meet the service demand and in fact has remained relatively stagnant over the past 30 years. Only recently has the number of US medical schools increased; however, the number of physicians graduated from the current complement of medical schools cannot meet the increased service demands, and will not be able to do so for the next several decades. This trend has led to an increase in offshore medical schools, particularly in the Caribbean region, where students complete their third and fourth years of clinical training and subsequently complete postgraduate training in US medical centers. Most of these students are American citizens who remain in practice in the United States.

In addition, many US medical school graduates have shifted from primary care—family medicine and general internal medicine—to the more lucrative medical and surgical specialties. The financial debt associated with US medical school education has been a main driver for the trend away from primary care specialization. The economics of the decision not to pursue specialization in this area is obvious: Primary care salaries are at the lower end of the professional compensation spectrum compared to their specialty counterparts. The US medical system historically has reimbursed specialty procedural skills well while poorly reimbursing the cognitive skill component of primary care practice.

The problem for physician leaders will be to determine how to meet the demand for primary care services to an increasing population in the presence of a major workforce shortage. International medical graduates have been filling the void in the total complement of US physicians. Will the deficit be fully remedied by utilizing mid-level providers or creating innovative financial incentives for US medical school graduates to enter primary care specialties? This is a critical issue facing physician leaders and will require a timely and sustainable solution.

## *Aging Population and End-of-Life Care*

Physician leaders are already confronted with an aging population. Baby boomers have entered the Medicare market and will be continuously joining this market for the next 15 years. The aging population in general will further burden the financial resources of an already constrained healthcare system. Medicare has begun reducing payments to healthcare systems in adherence to the value-based purchasing program, and increasing numbers of geriatric patients will merely multiply the financial deficits. Geriatricians, who have expertise in treating the maladies of the elderly, are not increasing in numbers commensurate with the increased number of elderly patients. Both family medicine and internal medicine residency training programs offer additional certificates of qualification in geriatric medicine to those board certified in the respective disciplines; however, the number of physicians pursuing this training will not be sufficient to meet the demand. How will healthcare systems deliver quality care to this expanding population? Physician leaders will have myriad issues to address with this population. Furthermore, the issues are expanding rapidly while the solutions are not readily apparent.

### Behavioral Health

Most large, established healthcare organizations in the United States, as well as many new systems, claim to offer healthcare integration as part of their mission. The extent to which they deliver on their integration claim depends on how they define the concept.

The World Health Organization (WHO) offers a comprehensive definition of integrated healthcare (Grone and Garcia-Barbero 2002):

> Integrated care is a concept bringing together inputs, delivery, management and organization of services related to diagnosis, treatment, care, rehabilitation and health promotion. Integration is a means to improve services in relation to access, quality, user satisfaction and efficiency.

The WHO definition clearly parallels the IHI Triple Aim in intent. However, some clinical areas in medicine remain orphans in the integrated model of care, most notably behavioral science and psychiatric care. These disciplines remain peripheral to considerations of the modern integrated healthcare system, which tends to include elements of a behavioral science system but lacks a comprehensive service.

Additional factors contributing to the absence of behavioral health in integrated care are the following:

- Healthcare insurers have historically provided limited coverage for these services.
- Psychiatrists are limited in number.
- Psychologists do not have prescriptive authority and must partner with a psychiatrist or primary care provider for those patients requiring psychotropic medication.

The system is not comprehensive and is clearly fragmented. How can any healthcare system boast integration in light of this contradiction?

Prevalence estimates of mental health disorders in the US adult population range from 20 to 25 percent. Untreated or inadequately treated mental health disorders are costly to individuals and to society. Psychiatric disorders have a tremendous impact on families (cost of care and emotional impact on family function), personal health (increased incidence of heart disease and cancer), personal well-being (disability), society (lost productivity, suicide), and the healthcare system (increased costs for poor reimbursement). Finally, although not as prevalent as one might believe from media accounts, inadequately treated patients with mental health issues have committed horrendous crimes.

Integrating psychiatric care and behavioral science into future healthcare reform will be a necessary and significant challenge for physician leaders. Traditional medical care generally subscribes to the medical model: recognition and treatment of defined disease states in which physicians focus on organ dysfunction and the treatment of that dysfunction. The biopsychosocial model of care integrates the disease in the context of many other factors, including psychological, social, cultural, and environmental. The traditional medical model has been historically well reimbursed by insurers while aspects of the biopsychosocial model frequently require the additional expertise of social workers, case managers, and others, which are not separately reimbursed by insurers but fall on the expense side of the healthcare organization.

The challenge for current and future physician leaders is to recognize and accept the fact that psychiatric disease treatment does not fit the mold of the medical model and falls into the category of the more complex biopsychosocial disease model. Leaders must further understand that the psychiatric disease burden is significant and undertreated, and their argument must convince insurers along with federal and state governments that an evolving, comprehensive plan for the treatment and reimbursement of psychiatric disease must be included in current and future discussions of national healthcare reform.

### Reimbursement and Bundled Payments

Medicare has launched a bundled payment initiative with orthopedic surgeons to reduce costs associated with total joint replacements (Mechanic 2015), and more bundled payment programs are expected. Physician leaders must be at the reimbursement table to ensure fairness of the disbursement to physicians while ensuring fiscal solvency for the healthcare system. Bundled payments will be a disruptive reimbursement system for physicians who are accustomed to the fee-for-service billings of the past century. Managing this change in physician payment structure will be a major challenge for physician leaders.

### Physician Unionization

As employment of medical providers increases, so will unionization. Physician unions have existed for decades throughout the European Union. In the United States, physician distrust of legislators, attorneys, hospitals, insurance companies, and healthcare executives makes the country a prime target for physician unionization.

Unionization of US physicians is not a new concept; it was first mentioned in the medical literature more than 50 years ago (Falk 1964). Unionization of medical providers could prove to be a major disruption to the US healthcare system.

## Telemedicine

Telemedicine was introduced in the United States several decades ago as a means to provide healthcare to patients in underserved rural areas. The technology has been developed and accepted as highly usable; however, the application of telemedicine has been stalled by insurers and federal and state governments. Many medical specialties, including psychiatry, dermatology, and cardiology, are amenable to telemedicine. Patients have demonstrated acceptance of the practice as a viable alternative to long-distance travel to see a physician, especially patients who live in rural areas. Physician leaders of the future have a distinct challenge to prove the worth of telemedicine to a wide set of stakeholders.

## Medical Consumerism and Medical Tourism

Medical consumerism and medical tourism may represent a boon for some health systems that are poised to cater to both phenomena, but their growth will bring increased concern for many physician leaders in the next decade. The ACA has helped define medical consumerism in the past few years, but to many consumers—as well as insurers—it has become anything but affordable. Many uninsured individuals have been able to secure medical insurance through the ACA's healthcare marketplace exchanges, but the cost of premiums is higher than many can easily manage and the deductibles are significant even with the best available insurance plans.

Another facet of consumerism in medicine is the wide availability of health applications at the consumer's fingertips via smartphones and tablet computers. Patients are able to manage their healthcare outside the physician office to greater efficacy than at any time in the past. Many apps are free or require a minimal financial investment. The alternative healthcare market is booming as well, with consumers eschewing primary care visits for acupuncture or other complementary treatments.

What impact will medical consumerism have on the finances of traditional medical care? Primarily, fewer visits will be made to medical providers and their organizations. Fewer visits leads to significant downstream consequences for healthcare systems in the form of fewer imaging studies, fewer laboratory studies, fewer referrals, and so on. Consumers may eventually utilize the traditional medical system only for significant illnesses.

Medical tourism poses a concern for the medical leadership establishment as well. Consumers can obtain modern healthcare in a variety of foreign countries for a fraction of the cost for the same care in the United States. And that care is not cheaper because it is delivered in dark alleys by medicine men and nontraditional practitioners. Instead, many countries that provide care to medical tourists offer it in sophisticated, well-appointed, state-of-the-art medical facilities staffed by physicians and surgeons who were trained in world-class medical centers in the United States and United Kingdom. Often, the cost for foreign healthcare, which includes the medical care, air transportation, and lodging, is significantly lower than the cost of medical care alone in the United States. Physician leaders will need to critically appraise the difference in costs for the same medical care between the United States and the countries offering medical tourism. Where can costs in the United States be trimmed to make care more affordable while assuring the public of high quality? This is just one question physicians must grapple with.

## *Disruptive Technologies and Disruptive Innovation*

Physician leaders must be vigilant for the emergence of disruptive technologies and disruptive innovation and their impact on traditional healthcare systems. One example of a disruptive innovation is the growth of retail clinics in large chains such as Wal-Mart, Target, and CVS pharmacies. These clinics provide low-cost, highly profitable medical services, such as the treatment of minor illnesses and immunizations, that are delivered by physician extenders. The convenient care offered by retail clinics is disruptive to existing healthcare systems because it is a low-cost alternative to the traditional appointment system. Retail clinics are popular with consumers, but historically, the healthcare profession has ignored patient access issues in favor of adhering to the appointment system, which results in higher costs, longer waits, and patient dissatisfaction. How will physician leaders cope with the loss of services and revenue to retail clinics? Offering similar services through physician extenders may be the immediate answer.

The EHR has clearly been the most disruptive technology in US medicine during the past decade. The technology was proposed as an integrative tool to store large volumes of retrievable patient data, a patient safety tool to eliminate prescribing errors, an advanced word processing tool to reduce documentation errors, a prescribing tool to reduce prescription errors and enhance patient safety, and a communication tool for medical providers across the continuum of healthcare. The EHR has thus far fallen short in many of these areas. In addition, it has been repeatedly cited as a contributing cause of physician burnout. Physician leaders must ensure that future EHR design and current EHR redesign efforts lead to provider-friendly features and enhance the practice of medicine rather than continue to be viewed by physicians as a time-consuming, sophisticated word processor.

Disruptive technologies will be commonplace in the future healthcare system. What will be the next disruptive technology to traditional healthcare? Could it be a smartphone application to manage diabetes by utilizing artificial intelligence implanted in a patient via a microchip? In a medical novel by Robin Cook (2014), this disruptive technological concept eliminated the traditional doctor–patient relationship in favor of protocol-driven medical care managed by artificial intelligence in the world of cyberspace. Fiction at present; reality in the not-too-distant future?

### *Quality and Patient Safety*

Patient safety remains an unhealed black eye for the US medical system, and physician leaders must be at the forefront of its solution. Physician leaders during the next decade will face a major moral and ethical crisis in quality and patient care, and they will need to heed the call to reduce medical errors to a benchmark that rivals the airline industry: less than 1 percent.

All these issues have contributed to the increasing recognition of the prevalence of physician burnout. To become a US physician has historically been an entry point into an elite and gratifying professional and social status. More recently, physicians have seen a significant and continuous erosion of their esteemed profession as multiple, evolving issues have chipped away at the professional status of the medical doctor. Most physicians' workload has increased with lower compensation; patient expectations and demands are high; federal and state governments are penalizing them for quality-of-care issues; costs of malpractice insurance have increased; and overall increased costs have forced physicians to abandon private practice and enter the world of traditional employment. Physicians feel a loss of control over their professional lives and destiny. They have become burned out and overwhelmed by work and increased stress and as a result are retiring early, reducing work hours, and encouraging their children to avoid a career in medicine. Physician suicide rates are now among the highest of any professional group (Andrew 2016; Schernhammer and Colditz 2004).

Physician leaders face a tremendous challenge regarding the growing physician burnout issue. The practice of medicine must be reinvented to be attractive for bright individuals and safe for the patients who require their care. Burnout must be eliminated to prevent deleterious effects on physicians and subsequently on their patients. One tenet of healthcare transformation is population management. The physician population in the United States was 916,264 in 2014 and estimated to increase by 12,168 annually in excess of physicians who retired or died. As of 2017, the projected physician population is approaching 1 million, at approximately 952,768 (Young et al. 2015).

This physician population carries an enormous responsibility to the public. Physician leaders must develop a new paradigm for the physician of the future by recognizing the wellness needs of physicians and balancing the professional role with work–life balance. This will be one of the greatest challenges for physician leadership and will require a multidisciplinary approach.

## Summary

The transformational changes that have already occurred and that continue to evolve in the US healthcare system demand effective physician leadership. Physicians who are educated in the principles of leadership must be able and willing to participate in healthcare decision making at all levels. No longer can medicine be led in silos. The business of medicine must be balanced by a healthcare system that provides high-quality care, timely patient access, and safety.

Chesley B. "Sully" Sullenberger, a former US Airways jet captain who made a remarkable emergency landing on the Hudson River in 2009 without losing a single passenger life, now frequently speaks publicly of medicine's failure to provide a high level of safety in patient care. He quotes the airline industries' crew resource management process, which ensures airline passenger safety at the 99th percentile, and contrasts it with the lack of standard operating procedures seen in the US healthcare system, which accepts as "safe" a healthcare environment scoring at the 90th percentile (Sullenberger 2013). Sullenberger asks, "Would the American public tolerate 10 percent of airline flights crashing daily?" The answer is obvious. Patient safety must be a primary focus of future physician leadership. Patient safety initiatives must be proactive and not reactive as they have been in the past. Medical risk management needs to be transformed into a high-reliability injury prevention system similar to that of the airline industry. Errors will occur in any system that depends on human judgment and behavior, but the margin of error in medical practice can be improved.

Much as a cardiac surgeon cannot perform complex heart surgery without extensive and exhaustive training, physicians cannot just desire to be leaders to become one. The physician leader who has already invested many years in medical education must be willing to invest additional time and financial resources to secure advanced leadership training while cascading through progressive leadership roles. This effort requires significant commitment on the part of aspiring physician leaders.

Physicians must learn and emulate the collaborative, responsive style of nonphysician leaders and administrators and abandon their individual, autocratic style. Physician leaders must define the moral imperative for the future healthcare system, and altruism must prevail in the reformed medical system, placing the patient at the center of that transformation. The US medical system must evolve into a high-quality delivery system with evidence-based treatments for the major diseases that affect diverse patient populations. Outcomes must be improved over the entire spectrum of disease.

Physicians in leadership roles must prove themselves worthy of the title. They must be judged and evaluated by established clinical outcome metrics while producing a financial margin in an era of cost containment and healthcare dollar constraint.

Physician executives must be at the forefront of visionary change and anticipate disruptive innovation. Medicine has for too long been reactionary to changes initiated by the federal government, healthcare insurers, big pharmacy, big business, and the legal system. Physician leaders must clearly lead and not just be content to game-manage a complex medical system.

The future of US medicine is here. Physician leaders must increase their influence by increasing their numbers. Leadership training should be introduced in the US medical school curriculum and postgraduate residency and fellowship training. In addition, the medical establishment must find a way to increase the number of practicing physicians—not to mention physicians entering leadership programs—in response to the projected need.

The case for physician leadership in modern healthcare has never been so clear; however, the challenges ahead for physician leaders are immense. Ultimately, the biggest challenge for physician leaders in the age of healthcare transformation will be to manage the change from a physician-centric culture to a patient-centered culture.

## Discussion Questions

1. Should physicians receive leadership training and take on leadership roles in the healthcare organization? Explain.
2. Should physicians actively participate in reinventing the healthcare system? If so, explain how they might do so.
3. Explain how the dyad model of healthcare leadership functions.
4. Describe in detail the many challenges physician leaders will face in the next decade.

## References

Andrew, L. B. 2016. "Physician Suicide." Medscape. Updated October 3. http://emedicine.medscape.com/article/806779-overview.

Angood, P., and S. Birk. 2014. "The Value of Physician Leadership." *Physician Executive* 40 (20): 1–16.

Barr, J., S. Bernard, S. Sofaer, T. Gianottii, N. Lenfestey, and D. Miranda. 2008. "Physicians' View on Public Reporting of Hospital Data." *Medical Care Research and Review* 65 (6): 655–73.

Berwick, D. M., T. W. Nolan, and J. Whittington. 2008. "The Triple Aim: Care, Health and Cost." *Health Affairs* 27 (3): 759–69.

Blendon, R., J. Benson, and J. Hero. 2014. "Public Trust in Physicians—U.S. Medicine in International Perspective." *New England Journal of Medicine* 371: 1570–72.

Brightman, B. 2007. "Medical Talent Management: A Model for Physician Deployment." *Leadership in Health Services* 20 (1): 27–32.

Cook, R. 2014. *Cell.* New York: Penguin.

Falk, I. S. 1964. "Labor Unions and Medical Care." *New England Journal of Medicine* 270: 22–28.

Farrell, J. P., and M. M. Robbins. 1993. "Leadership Competencies for Physicians." *Healthcare Forum Journal* 36 (4): 39–42.

Frontain, M. 2017. "Enron Corporation." *Handbook of Texas Online.* Updated February 9. www.tshaonline.org/handbook/online/articles/doe08.

Gallup. 2016. "Honesty/Ethics in Professions." Polling of December 7–11. www.gallup.com/poll/171710/public-faith-congree-falls-again-hits-historic-low.aspx.

Goodall, A. 2011. "Physician Leaders and Hospital Performance: Is There an Association?" *Social Science and Medicine* 73 (4): 535–39.

Grone, O., and M. Garcia-Barbero. 2002. *Trends in Integrated Care—Reflections on Conceptual Issues.* Copenhagen, Denmark: World Health Organization.

Institute for Healthcare Improvement (IHI). 2016. "The IHI Triple Aim." Accessed December 26. www.ihi.org/engage/initiatives/tripleaim/pages/default.aspx.

McKenna, M. K., M. P. Gartland, and P. A. Pugno. 2004. "Development of Physician Leadership Competencies: Perceptions of Physician Leaders, Physician Educators and Medical Students." *Journal of Health Administration Education* 21: 343–54.

Mechanic, R. E. 2015. "Mandatory Medicare Bundled Payment—Is It Ready for Prime Time?" *New England Journal of Medicine* 373: 1291–93.

Olivo, T. 2014. "The Profile of an Effective Healthcare Leader." *Becker's Hospital Review.* Published March 11. www.beckershospitalreview.com/hospital-management-administration/the-profile-of-an-effective-healthcare-leader.html.

Satiani, B., J. Sena, R. Ruberg, and E. C. Ellison. 2014. "Talent Management and Physician Leadership Training Is Essential for Preparing Tomorrow's Physician Leaders." *Journal of Vascular Surgery* 59 (2): 542–46.

Schernhammer, E., and G. Colditz. 2004. "Suicide Rates Among Physicians: A Quantitative and Gender Assessment (Meta-analysis)." *American Journal of Psychiatry* 161: 2295–302.

Stoller, J. K. 2008. "Developing Physician-Leaders: Key Competencies and Available Programs." *Journal of Health Administration Education* 25 (4): 307–29.

Sullenberger, C. 2013. "Aviation and Medical Errors." Presentation to the American Medical Group Association Annual Conference, Orlando, Florida, March 16.

Young, A., H. Chaudhry, X. Pei, K. Halbesleben, D. Polk, and M. Dugan. 2015. "A Census of Actively Licensed Physicians in the United States, 2014." *Journal of Medical Regulation* 101 (2): 1–22.

Zismer, D., and J. Brueggeman. 2010. "Examining the Dyad as a Management Model in Integrated Health Systems." *Physician Executive* 36: 14–19.

# LEADERSHIP CASE STUDIES

This section of the book contains five case studies used to demonstrate some of the key concepts presented in the text. They are designed to promote thoughtful consideration and responses rather than straightforward solutions.

After reading each case study, answer the questions by using the following method:

- Clarify the facts in the case.
- Define the problem, not the symptoms of the problem.
- Identify potential solutions to the problem identified.
- Develop a solution implementation plan.
- Develop an evaluation process for the proposed solution.
- Either individually or as a group, write a group response to the questions posed at the end of each case.

## CASE STUDY 1

# LEADERSHIP AND NEVER EVENTS

Bernard J. Healey

In its landmark study *To Err Is Human,* the Institute of Medicine (2000) estimated that from 44,000 to 98,000 of the 33 million individual patients hospitalized every year die, and many more contract hospital-acquired infections. These types of medical mistakes are often referred to as "never events" because they can be prevented and thus should never occur. The major reason offered by medical researchers for these errors is a lack of communication or poor communication among providers of care. Patients commonly receive medical care from numerous providers, and in many cases, some of those providers do not have accurate and up-to-date medical information about their patients. This lack of information often leads to medication errors.

The CEO of hospital A, John Dawson, is faced with his second outbreak of methicillin-resistant *Staphylococcus aureus* (MRSA) in three weeks. Meeting with the hospital's infection control nurse, Betty McGuire, and chief of medical services, Dr. Malone, Dawson is visibly upset. McGuire reports that over the past three weeks, 27 cases of MRSA occurred on two floors of the six-story hospital.

Fortunately, the organization has in place a superb active surveillance system for communicable diseases, so a great deal of information is available to leaders concerning the MRSA infections. The confirmed cases of MRSA have been isolated from the hospital's general population, and the local public health department has been notified of the outbreak. The epidemiologist from the county health department has already begun conducting a case control study. However, Dawson is concerned that MRSA is not being prevented, causing patients undue discomfort and increasing costs to both patients and the hospital.

The CEO's meetings with this group have been taking place for the past week in an attempt to keep stakeholders informed about the MRSA outbreak. Dawson has appointed McGuire as the chief spokesperson regarding the disease outbreak and has been keeping the local media informed about the problem. The local health department continues to submit samples to the laboratory and reports no additional

*(continued)*

*(continued from previous page)*

cases for two maximum incubation periods. The health department also has informed Dawson that it is pleased with the control measures put in place by the hospital.

Though staff and leaders have taken all the appropriate steps in response to the second outbreak, the CEO and medical director state that they will not be happy until they find out what caused the outbreak and know how to prevent future outbreaks at the hospital. They request that McGuire continue the investigation until she is satisfied that the mode of transmission of MRSA is discovered. They also ask her to prepare an honest critique of the control measures administered by the hospital. Once this information is gathered, the group plans to meet to craft a written proposal for all staff in the hospital to follow for preventing future outbreaks.

## QUESTIONS

1. What was the underlying cause of this hospital-acquired outbreak of disease? How could it have been prevented?
2. How can the surveillance system currently in use by this hospital be improved to provide early warnings to the CEO?
3. Once the final report on this hospital-acquired disease outbreak is completed, who should receive copies of the report? Explain your reasons for sharing this report with these individuals.

## REFERENCE

Institute of Medicine. 2000. *To Err Is Human: Building a Safer Health System.* Washington, DC: National Academies Press.

## CASE STUDY 2

# LEADERSHIP IN WELLNESS PROGRAMS

Susan Diana and Dana Abend

Emanuel (2014) points out that costs continue to rise while quality of care continues to diminish on an annual basis. Strategies such as higher deductibles, increased copayments, and larger employee premiums are being implemented to decrease employers' healthcare costs. The weakness of these strategies is the focus on cost containment directly rather than addressing the core problem of unhealthy lifestyles leading to chronic disease.

In response to this issue, employers should create wellness programs that stress prevention to eliminate the high cost of chronic disease management. Such programs offer monetary incentives to employees to make healthful lifestyle changes that will positively affect their health and eventually lower healthcare spending as well as increase productivity and morale. No gold standard exists for creating a worksite wellness program; however, the following review of the literature offers several approaches to a successful wellness program.

Kaspin, Gorman, and Miller (2013) analyzed research from studies conducted between 2004 and 2009 looking at 20 enduring employer-sponsored worksite wellness programs to determine what factors have rendered them successful over time. The companies were diverse in their business lines, but all supported worksite wellness programs for their employees.

Researchers categorized interventions into three areas: health risk assessments, lifestyle management programs, and behavioral health programs. The outcomes were defined as economic, clinical, or patient related. Economic outcomes were divided into direct (cost savings or return on investment [ROI], healthcare utilization) or indirect (absenteeism, presentism, productivity, workers' compensation). Health-related outcomes included patients' view of their quality of life, changes in health risk factors, or the practice of health behaviors (improvements in exercise or eating habits). Many of the companies studied offered monetary incentives in the form of cash or gift cards to employees to participate in worksite wellness programs. Other incentives offered were reductions in health insurance premiums and

*(continued)*

*(continued from previous page)*

medication costs for employees who participated and were able to lower their health risks.

The average annual savings per employee was $565. In addition, those companies that offered wellness programs experienced a lower rate of increase in their direct healthcare costs or a decrease in those costs over time.

Tobacco cessation, increased exercise, and risk reduction were the three most common health-related outcomes reported from the studies reviewed. Employees tended to experience improved health and well-being, which led to lowered absenteeism. One of the companies, Con-way Freight, reported an increase in the number of employees who exercise at least twice a week for 20 minutes in the first year of the program, which resulted in weight loss for 831 employees totaling 626 pounds.

The companies that had reported positive outcomes in their wellness programs all shared many qualities. Achieving a positive ROI from wellness programs can take several years to manifest, and the companies that experienced a positive return shared an optimistic outlook for their wellness program at the outset, with support starting at the top of the company and trickling down to department heads and then to all staff. The culture in these companies is one of positive health, with the goal of living an enhanced life, not just an improved corporate bottom line. As part of this culture-building process, some companies extended their wellness programs to include the spouses and children of employees. Others established walking paths, built on-site gyms, or offered fitness classes scheduled around business hours. Over time, as the environment changed, so did the design of the programs to support the needs of the company and the employees.

When implementing a wellness program, an intake process needs to be established to set benchmarks by which to measure outcomes. To capture this information, organizations should have in place a clinical decision support system (CDSS). Amirfar and colleagues (2011) summarized different outcomes of the development and implementation of a CDSS achieved through an initiative of the New York City Department of Health and Mental Hygiene called Take Care New York. By reviewing the process undergone by the Primary Care Information Project (PCIP), Amirfar and his team offered recommendations that

*(continued)*

*(continued from previous page)*

could lead to enhancements in future CDSS builds. The goal of PCIP was to create a system to improve the health of the people in New York City by creating a system focused on ten healthcare measures.

The government worked with the vendor of its electronic health record system (EHR) to include quality measures that prompted providers to encourage preventive care or chronic disease management pending assessment of the patient's health status. Any organization embarking on development of an EHR must ensure that its communication between healthcare staff and technical staff is clear and continuous. PCIP found that in the collaboration process the facts were well understood by both parties, but that level of mutual understanding did not occur in the translation of the clinical measures to the computer program. Once PCIP was developed, staff discovered they had underestimated the time and effort required for the testing phase to discover and fix errors that resulted from the misunderstandings.

The following recommendations were made by Amirfar and colleagues (2011) for future endeavors in building a CDSS within an EHR:

1. Define the scope of the project and obtain agreement on it from all parties involved with support from executive leadership.
2. Select software partners that are enthusiastic about and share the vision for the project.
3. Have a clear operational strategy with constant communication between clinicians and developers.
4. Test the system with real-world scenarios to ensure that the system works correctly for its users.
5. Seek assistance from those who have already undergone the CDSS build process and were successful.

In the end, if a CDSS is implemented successfully, the health outcomes desired will be more attainable than if the CDSS implementation encounters problems or ultimately fails.

## QUESTIONS

1. Explain the value of wellness programs being added as an employee benefit.

*(continued)*

*(continued from previous page)*

2. What role can be played by an electronic health record system in the prevention of chronic diseases and their complications? Explain.

## REFERENCES

Amirfar, S., J. Taverna, S. Anane, and J. Singer. 2011. "Developing Public Health Clinical Decision Support Systems (CDSS) for the Outpatient Community in New York City: Our Experience." *BMC Public Health* 11 (1): 753.

Emanuel, E. 2014. *Reinventing American Healthcare: How the Affordable Care Act Will Improve Our Terribly Complex, Blatantly Unjust, Grossly Inefficient, Error Prone System*. New York: Public Affairs.

Kaspin, L. C., K. M. Gorman, and R. M. Miller. 2013. "Systematic Review of Employer-Sponsored Wellness Strategies and their Economic and Health-Related Outcomes." *Population Health Management* 16 (1): 14–21.

CASE STUDY 3

# #ThinkBeforeYouPost

Katie P. Desiderio

Ella changed the privacy settings on her Facebook account to the most secure option, just as her nursing professor advised. While she understood the importance of being cautious, she thought the nursing faculty members were taking social media privacy to a new level of vigilance. "I've had it with lectures on using social media responsibly; seriously, what can really happen?" Ella wondered. Before she could continue venting online to her friend Grayce, her professor interrupted. "Ella, please put your phone away during class, and this request is extended to the rest of the class, too. The obsession with your cell phones has got to stop, people!" Ella rolled her eyes at Professor Cole's comment and gazed off for the remainder of the class.

*(continued)*

*(continued from previous page)*

At the close of the third quarter of 2015, Facebook reported 1.55 billion active users (Statista 2017). Furthermore, Mark Zuckerberg (2015), founder of Facebook, noted that "for the first time ever [on August 27, 2015], one billion people used Facebook in a single day." The nursing faculty members at Ella's nursing school are theoretically aware of the implications pertaining to responsible usage of social media; conversely, many don't use this medium, so the learning curve is reciprocally influential for both faculty and students. St. Isabelle's Hospital, the primary partner of the nursing program, has encouraged the college to proactively provide supplementary reading to students on the ethical responsibilities of nursing staff; guidelines for using social media; and, of course, awareness of the Health Insurance Portability and Accountability Act of 1996 (HIPAA). The hospital's stance is that, considering the severity of a breach in patient confidentiality, technology has certainly changed accessibility to patient protected information for anyone working in healthcare. The Office for Civil Rights of the US Department of Health & Human Services (2015) enforces

> the HIPAA Privacy Rule, which protects the privacy of individually iden-
> tifiable health information; the HIPAA Security Rule, which sets national
> standards for the security of electronic protected health information; the
> HIPAA Breach Notification Rule, which requires covered entities and busi-
> ness associates to provide notification following a breach of unsecured pro-
> tected health information; and the confidentiality provisions of the Patient
> Safety Rule, which protect identifiable information being used to analyze
> patient safety events and improve patient safety.

As a tenured faculty member and chair of the nursing program, Professor John Cole had never anticipated just how much technology would affect his work. With a new awareness, he became acclimated with the issue by reading the first recommended resource, from *The Online Journal of Issues in Nursing*'s 2012 publication "Guidelines for Using Electronic and Social Media: The Regulatory Perspective," before assigning it to students. He was struck by a segment in the first few paragraphs that read, "participating in social media is not a problem as long as nurses always remain cognizant of their professional obligations" (Spector and Kappel 2012). Cole read the statement again, reflecting on how it applied to every member of his department, from

*(continued)*

*(continued from previous page)*

faculty to staff to students. As he finished the article, he began thinking about the ways he would integrate its guidance into his courses.

Cole then searched for definitions of social media. He found that Kaplan and Haenlein (2010, 61) define social media as "a group of Internet-based applications that build on the ideological and technological foundations of Web 2.0, and that allow the creation and exchange of user-generated content." For another perspective pertaining specifically to the nursing profession, according to Bulman and Schutz (2008), social media is "an outlet where nurses can share workplace experiences, particularly those events that are challenging, [that] can be as invaluable as journaling and reflective practice, which have been identified as effective tools in nursing practice." To maintain the college's treasured partnership with St. Isabelle's Hospital and the overall credibility of the nursing program, Cole realized that explicit educational opportunities surrounding HIPAA and social media consumption must be woven into the curriculum. As he thought about the exciting, and daunting, learning opportunities, Cole sat back in his chair and enjoyed the glistening of the sun leaving a rainbow across his desk. His calming thoughts were interrupted by an insistent knock on his door. "John, we have a big problem that needs our attention. Now."

As a senior in the nursing program, Ella was enjoying her clinical rotations and felt eager to begin her career in nursing. She was especially excited about the opportunity to learn more in the obstetrics and gynecology department of St. Isabelle's, where she had been spending every Tuesday since the start of the semester. She had never considered the extent of this specialty, nor had she anticipated the wide range of exposure to everything from reproductive cysts to the variety of birthing methods. It was nearly 11:30 a.m., and the patient in room 205 would be arriving soon following recovery from her scheduled cesarean section. Ella decided to use her few minutes of downtime to check Facebook before her day grew busy again. "Oh YAY, this is so exciting," Ella squealed, forgetting where she was. She quickly "liked" Grayce's recent post that their favorite professor was expecting a baby in May. "Wow," Ella thought, "a baby. Professor Lee must be so thrilled!" A smile formed across her face at the thought of her professor as a mom; she couldn't wait to congratulate her on campus tomorrow!

When Ella left the hospital that evening, she texted Grayce, excited to learn more about Professor Lee's pregnancy announcement. This text message exchange followed:

*(continued)*

*(continued from previous page)*

> *Ella*: Hey, hey pretty! ♥ Saw your FB post about Lee . . . soooo excited!! ☺
> How did u find out?! What is she having?
>
> *Grayce* [responded immediately]: I knowww, can u believe it?! ♥♥ She came
> in today for an ultrasound and seemed as surprised as us. I really hope we
> can babysit!!♥

The blood drained from Ella's face and her excitement dissolved; she felt nauseous. She could hear Professor Cole's voice in her mind saying, "As aspiring nurses, you must consider how and when to use social media. THINK before you post." Grayce sent another text, "u there?" Ella began typing, but couldn't formulate her thoughts. She resorted to, "call when u can talk." Ella's phone rang moments later.

Back on campus, Cole was frantically gathering information about the college's policy for handling such a breach of privacy. He knew he also had to consider the hospital's policy as noted in its partnership agreement with the nursing program. While he was gratified that his colleague alerted him to Grayce's Facebook post, he recognized he had more to learn about the privacy, or lack thereof, of social media. He was unaware that liking a post appears on the newsfeed of that friend for anyone to see. His mind was racing with what to do first. In his 20 years in higher education, he never imagined he would be considering expulsion for a student's misuse of social media. Is expelling Grayce too harsh? Will the nursing program be legally liable for sharing personal patient (and faculty) information without consent? Will Ella face any consequences for liking the post? Does Ella realize that when you like a post, it is shared to your Facebook newsfeed? Does the college have a current social media policy in place? Cole had so many implications to consider. He needed to consult with the college's provost before making any decisions, but first he had to get in touch with Grayce to have her delete her post. Questions continued to flood his mind.

## QUESTIONS

1. Offer a comprehensive definition of social media.
2. Will the nursing program be legally liable for sharing personal patient (and faculty) information without consent?
3. What is the most important lesson to be learned from this case study?

*(continued)*

*(continued from previous page)*

**REFERENCES**

Bulman, C., and S. Schutz (eds.). 2008. *Reflective Practice in Nursing.* Hoboken, NJ: Wiley-Blackwell.

Kaplan, A. M., and M. Haenlein. 2010. "Users of the World, Unite! The Challenges and Opportunities of Social Media." *Business Horizons* 53 (1): 59–68.

Spector, N., and D. Kappel. 2012. "Guidelines for Using Electronic and Social Media: The Regulatory Perspective." *OJIN: The Online Journal of Issues in Nursing.* Published September 30. www.nursing world.org/MainMenuCategories/ANAMarketplace/ANAPeriodicals /OJIN/TableofContents/Vol-17-2012/No3-Sept-2012/Guidelines-for -Electronic-and-Social-Media.html.

Statista. 2017. *Numbers of Active Facebook Users Worldwide as of 3rd Quarter 2015.* Accessed January 13. www.statista.com/statistics /264810/number-of-monthly-active-facebook-users-worldwide/.

US Department of Health & Human Services. 2015. "Health Information Privacy." Accessed January 13, 2017. www.hhs.gov/ocr/privacy/.

Zuckerberg, M. 2015. Facebook post. August 27. www.facebook.com /zuck/posts/10102329188394581.

CASE STUDY 4

# LEADERSHIP IN A CHANGING HEALTHCARE ENVIRONMENT

Bernard J. Healey

The CEO of healthcare system X, Marcus Williams, is faced with declining revenues, decreases in quality of care, and the departure of several key leaders. He feels the entire workforce has become reluctant to use its individual creativity in the design of innovations that are so necessary in the changing environment the organization faces. Williams has taken several leadership courses and done a fair amount of reading about leadership and its role in getting an organization prepared to

*(continued)*

*(continued from previous page)*

respond to extreme change. From these readings, Williams has come to believe he must get his entire workforce involved in innovation to improve the healthcare facilities' finances along with the quality of services delivered to consumers.

Williams starts this process by holding a meeting with two of the system's vice presidents, Gloria Adams and Shawn McGroarty. The purpose of the meeting is for the CEO to explain the importance of getting everyone working together to design a creative approach to solving the system's current problems. Williams asks the vice presidents to survey their managers about their interest in participating in focus groups regarding the financial and quality issues and the development of some potential solutions. It seems that every sector of the healthcare industry is being disrupted by start-up businesses seeking to make a profit from the enormous change occurring in healthcare services delivery. In fact, much of the current research supports the notion that if you are not innovating, you are likely not going to be a viable business in the long-term.

One of the most difficult areas of concern for leaders in healthcare today is to get their facilities and employees to understand the need for change in the way they do business. Over the next few years, almost every aspect of the delivery of healthcare services is likely to change. Most individuals fear change and do not understand why healthcare organizations have a need to change. Despite the desire by organizations and employees to resist change, a tremendous amount of evidence suggests that the pace of change in the healthcare environment is already accelerating rapidly. These changes in healthcare delivery will require empowered and motivated employees capable of delivering superior services on a daily basis.

## Questions

1. What are some additional concerns that the CEO should express to his vice presidents at the first meeting regarding the current problems being faced by the healthcare organization?

2. Would a leadership training program be helpful for all the employees of this healthcare organization to spur them to innovate? What areas of training should be included if such a program were offered to staff?

CASE STUDY 5

# Transforming Community Health

Justin Beaupre

Donita Murphy is a primary care physician at a local community practice clinic. She was recently asked to consult with the local health department to help develop programs that will improve the health of community residents. In the past decade, community organizations, health departments, and healthcare systems have begun to transform and reevaluate health and healthcare. A significant rise in the cost of healthcare services has community health leaders focused on the importance of health promotion programs that engage community members to participate in programs that will foster a culture of health. Affordability and quality care should be synonymous as community health leaders determine ways to provide preventive health services to the local community.

At the first meeting with health department leaders, Murphy listened intently as officials discussed what they believed to be the most serious health disparities and concerns in the community. Some of the responses included a recent rise in crime rates, obesity, smoking, diabetes, substance and drug abuse, poverty, and lack of funding for services. After a half hour of discussion, no one had yet asked Murphy, a physician who has been treating residents for nearly 30 years, what she thought about the health of the community. When she finally had the chance to speak, she asked everyone in the room several questions, to which none of the other attendees had clear answers:

1. What do the residents of this community feel are the most important factors positively or negatively affecting health?
2. How do you perceive or value your own health? What does health mean to you, and what experiences have shaped your interpretation of health?
3. How does community leadership support improving the quality of health?

Murphy's patients are predominantly residents of low-income housing, receiving financial assistance for medical care government

*(continued)*

(continued from previous page)

subsidies to support the cost of living. They have struggled to find employment in a community that has seen factories close and companies outsource. She has witnessed firsthand the daily struggles of residents to afford quality care; access preventive health; participate in health and wellness activities; improve their education and job skills; and afford fresh, healthful food.

Murphy believes community health leaders who wish to change the culture of health should use their knowledge and education to influence change by teaching people the value of health, providing them with the knowledge and tools to make informed decisions regarding health and health behaviors, and providing an avenue for educational and economic opportunities to better health. Transformative leadership focuses on "the ability of the leader to reach the souls of others in a fashion which raises human consciousness, builds meanings, and inspires human intent that is the source of power" (Bennis 1986, 70). In underserved communities, the barriers to better health are often caused by a lack of shared power between leadership and residents to create change and influence policies that can help redistribute health resources. Community health leaders, therefore, should collaborate with residents to build strong community organizations that will implement health promotion programs, empower people who have felt powerless, and identify health inequities and inequalities. Improving the health of a community requires an investment from residents, the healthcare delivery system, local businesses, and community leaders. Murphy contends that communities that work together to create a shared vision, identify issues that have created inequity and inequality, and identify local resources that may help provide solutions to improve health conditions within the community will see the greatest health improvements.

The local health network was recently purchased by a for-profit company, leaving many residents unable to afford or access healthcare services. They rely on the local health department to offer health services. A significant reduction in the health department's budget is making it even more difficult for community health leaders to provide necessary services. Murphy suggests that the health department be proactive, rather than reactive, in understanding the health concerns in the community, encouraging community collaboration to improve health, and meeting with residents to identify health inequities and the impact those gaps have on health.

(continued)

*(continued from previous page)*

## QUESTIONS

1. Why are the questions posed by Donita Murphy essential to transforming community health?
2. How do the recent changes in the socioeconomic status of the community affect health disparities?
3. Viewing the situation through a transformative lens, how can community health leaders work with residents, businesses, and the local healthcare system to change the conditions in which people live, work, and grow?

## REFERENCE

Bennis, W. 1986. "Transformative Power and Leadership." In *Leadership and Organizational Culture: New Perspectives on Administrative Theory and Practice,* edited by T. J. Sergiovanni and J. E. Corbally, 64–71. Champaign, IL: University of Illinois Press.

# GLOSSARY

**Administrative model**. An approach to leadership that relies on a nonmedical healthcare manager for efficiency.

**Affordable Care Act (ACA)**. Signed into law in 2010, the act seeks to increase the quality and availability of healthcare coverage for most Americans.

**American Association for Physician Leadership**. A professional association that focuses on training and supporting physicians to hold hospital and health system leadership positions.

**Authentic**. Demonstrating genuine characteristics to others at all times, thereby showing worthiness of their trust.

**Biomedical entrepreneurship**. Activity that produces new medical devices, drugs, and medical treatments.

**Bonding**. The building of a sense of community among employees.

**Breach of trust**. Failure to act in a way that is expected based on confidence in and reliance on the actor.

**Bundled payment system**. A reimbursement structure by which a single payment is made to two or more physicians for a particular episode of care.

**Bureaucratic organization**. A corporate structure that focuses on rules and regulations to achieve efficiency.

**Capitation**. A payment scheme by which a provider of healthcare is paid a set amount to deliver care for a certain period.

**Change management**. The thoughtful identification and implementation of new ways to accomplish goals.

**Charisma**. The compelling attractiveness or charm of an individual that affords the individual personal power.

**Charismatic skill**. Attractiveness and charm that can lead to devotion by others.

**Climate**. The attitude that workers have regarding the work they do and the organization they perform that work for.

**Cognitive response**. The set of thoughts or silent personal self-talk that occurs during an interaction.

**Comparative effectiveness research (CER)**. Studies that evaluate the benefits, harms, and effectiveness of different treatment options.

**Conflict**. A serious and upsetting disagreement or argument between two or more individuals, typically over clashes in opinion, values, or actions.

**Conflict management**. The concept that discord or disagreement can be helpful for growth but needs to be managed.

**Conflict management style**. The way a leader handles situations of discord.

**Contingency theory**. Theory that states there is no best way to organize an organization.

**Continuous quality improvement**. An approach to quality in which managers and workers continually strive for improved performance.

**Cost–benefit analysis**. An economics-focused process for comparing the strengths and weaknesses of alternative choices in healthcare provision.

**Cost-effectiveness analysis**. An economics-focused process for comparing the cost of an intervention to its effectiveness.

**Creative destruction**. The use of capital resources to devise a product or service that is more valuable than the original capital.

**Creativity**. The ability to create something new and valuable.

**Culture**. A way of thinking or behaving in an organization.

**Culture audit**. A formal investigation of the culture of an organization.

**Culture building**. The leader's activities related to creating a strong working climate for employees.

**Design thinking**. A method for designing new human-centered products and services.

**Digital support system**. Suite of applications that work in conjunction with electronic health records.

**Disruptive innovation**. A new way of operating that typically begins in smaller companies and diffuses throughout an industry, causing upheaval to other businesses in that industry.

**Dual operating system**. A structure for running a business under parallel schemes that feature the creativity of a start-up and the efficiencies of a mature business.

**Dyad model**. An approach to leadership in which the physician leader and administrative leader work together in distinct but complementary roles.

**Emotional intelligence**. The ability to have a keen awareness of others' emotions and to effectively express and control one's own emotions when dealing with others.

**Empowerment**. The freedom conferred by management on lower-level employees to make decisions without asking for permission.

**Entrepreneurial innovation**. Consists of new ways to innovate resulting in greater wealth creation.

**Entrepreneurial success**. The extent to which an individual is effective in the process of wealth creation.

**Entrepreneurship**. A way of creating wealth with a new business innovation.

**Fee-for-service**. A healthcare services reimbursement model whereby providers are paid for the quantity of services offered.

**Flow**. A mental state in which work is enjoyable, challenging, and ultimately productive.

**Health education programs**. Teaching strategies and tools designed to develop awareness in the population about good and bad health behaviors.

**Human capital**. The collective skills and knowledge of the workforce, including creativity brought by employees to the organization to create value.

**Hybrid educational model**. Combines a traditional face-to-face class with outside classroom experiences.

**Illness system**. An approach to care delivery that focuses on illness rather than wellness.

**Informal leader**. An individual who has developed power without being an appointed manager.

**Innovation**. The creation of new or improved products or services.

**Innovation approach**. A method of designing new, increasingly efficient ways of delivering healthcare to patients.

**Institute for Healthcare Improvement (IHI)**. Organization dedicated to improving healthcare services worldwide.

**Integrated healthcare system**. An organizational arrangement that focuses on the coordination of patient care.

**Integrity**. The consistent demonstration of honesty and strong moral principles.

**Intermediary**. An individual or organization that works between a buyer and a seller of a product or service.

**Internal culture**. The values and beliefs of a business that are found deep within the organization.

**Internship**. On-the-job training that may be offered by a college for academic credit.

**Interpersonal skills**. Qualities that involve getting along with people.

**Interpersonal conflict**. Discord between two or more individuals.

**Intrinsic motivation**. Impetus to act found within the individual and driven by internal rewards.

**Involuntary trust**. A default state of trust that is created between two parties in light of a power imbalance and the necessity of dependency of one party on the other party for care.

**Leadership development**. A series of educational programs designed to facilitate the growth of leadership traits in individuals.

**Learning organization**. An entity that places great value on the constant growth of employees in terms of education and training.

**Least-preferred coworker (LPC) scale**. Theory that considers the concept of a fellow employee with whom others prefer not to work on a project.

**Legacy**. The qualities and values that one will be remembered for in one's work.

**Managed care**. Techniques adopted by third-party payers to reduce the cost and improve the quality of healthcare.

**Management development**. Training programs that assist managers in job improvement.

**Mission statement**. A formal document to explain an organization's core goals and values.

**MRSA (methicillin-resistant *Staphylococcus aureus*)**. A type of staph bacteria that has become resistant to antibiotics.

**Needs assessment**. A method of determining and prioritizing what individuals need to learn.

**Network structure**. A type of operational framework in which employees are empowered to pursue new products or ways of delivering services.

**Organizational life cycle**. The distinct stages of an organization's growth and decline.

**Organizational structure**. The way activities and positions are organized toward the accomplishment of goals.

**Paradigm**. A pattern or system of how activities are performed to ensure successful completion.

**Paradigm shift**. A change in the way one thinks about how to proceed through a process or design an activity.

**Passive resistance**. Noncompliance with authority; differentiated from active resistance by ignoring authority and not cooperating with requests for change.

**Patient-centered healthcare**. The provision of health services in a manner that is respectful of the patient's desires and expectations as well as clinical needs.

**Patient-centered medical home (PCMH)**. A care delivery model in which healthcare is provided and coordinated through a primary care doctor.

**Pay-for-performance (P4P)**. A payment system that offers providers of care financial incentives for achieving improved patient outcomes.

**Perception**. The way an individual views the world.

**Performance standard**. A time-bound objective for an employee.

**Phase-gate process**. A way to divide a process into steps that move from idea to implementation.

**Physiological response**. An automatic, instinctive response to a stressful situation manifesting in observable physical markers such as heightened blood pressure, heart rate, muscle tension, and a change in breathing patterns.

**Power base**. A foundation of authority, whether given by the organization or owned by the individual, that secures the right to lead.

**Price sensitivity**. An estimate of how much a consumer will change the quantity purchased of a good or service based on a change in price for that good or service.

**Primary conflict tension**. The stress produced by the initial conflict.

**Productivity.** The level of output related to input.

**Psychological trap.** A management barrier to progress that occurs when an organization holds on to the past as the default option.

**Reinvention.** The activity of making major changes and improvements.

**Resource trap.** A situation prohibitive to growth in which organizations invest scarce resources in old systems that do not work.

**Results pyramid.** A model of culture change that concentrates on the most important parts of the organization.

**Scientific management.** The theory of studying work processes to increase productivity.

**Self-efficacy.** The belief of individuals in whether they can or cannot accomplish a goal or perform an activity.

**Sense of urgency.** A belief, evident in one's behavior, that action must be taken immediately.

**Servant leadership.** Style of leadership that occurs when serving and leading are in harmony.

**Six Sigma.** A data-driven approach to eliminating defects that sets as a standard no more than six errors per 1 million opportunities (the statistical threshold of $6\sigma$).

**Sociopathy.** Antisocial behavior characterized by a lack of a sense of moral responsibility and lack of good conscience.

**Sources of power.** Rewards, punishment, legitimacy, expertise, and referent.

**Stewardship.** The responsible management of scarce resources.

**Subculture.** A part of an organization that holds some beliefs that vary from those of the parent culture.

**Technological enabler.** An advancement in the way things have been done in the past.

**10X companies.** Business entities that have achieved superior growth over time, by a factor of ten over their counterparts.

**Thick positive culture.** A working climate that supports excellence and is widespread throughout the organization.

**Trust.** A feeling that connotes honesty and reliability.

**Turbulence.** A state of chaotic occurrences causing unpredictable change.

**Value proposition.** A belief that the proposed change will present benefits to the consumer.

# INDEX

Note: Italicized page locators refer to figures or tables in exhibits.

# ABOUT THE AUTHOR

**Bernard J. Healey, PhD,** is a professor of healthcare administration at King's College in Wilkes-Barre, Pennsylvania. Dr. Healey began his career in 1971 as an epidemiologist for the Pennsylvania Department of Health. During his tenure with the government, he earned his master's in public administration and his doctorate in health education from the University of Pennsylvania. He has taught undergraduate and graduate courses in business, public health, and healthcare administration at several colleges since 1974. He has coauthored five books on healthcare topics and has published more than a hundred articles on public health, health policy, leadership, marketing, and healthcare partnerships. Dr. Healey is a member of the American Public Health Association and of the Association of University Programs in Health Administration. He is a part-time consultant in epidemiology for the Wilkes-Barre City Health Department and a consultant for numerous public health projects in Pennsylvania.

# ABOUT THE CONTRIBUTORS

The numerous contributors to this new text were generous enough to share their expertise of healthcare in the form of chapters or case studies. These contributors include the following individuals.

**Tina Marie Evans** is associate professor and department head of applied health studies at Pennsylvania College of Technology. A 1998 summa cum laude graduate of Marywood University with a bachelor's degree in sports medicine, she has a master's of healthcare administration degree from King's College and a doctorate in health promotion from Marywood University. She is active in grant writing; publishing scholarly manuscripts; and presenting on various allied health topics on the local, regional, national, and international levels. Evans also continues to volunteer for her church and community and enjoys the outdoors, swimming, golf, ballroom dancing, and spending time with her family.

**Nancy Sayre, DHEd**, is chair of the health professions department in the College of Professional Studies at Metropolitan State University of Denver. She has taught courses in entrepreneurship, leadership, and management in the healthcare industry and has led efforts to develop new university courses and programs. Previously, she worked as a consultant and executive in a variety of healthcare corporations, assisting them in developing successful products and generating new business development opportunities.

**Jeffrey Helton, PhD, FHFMA**, is assistant professor of healthcare management at Metropolitan State University of Denver, where he teaches healthcare finance, health informatics, and health economics. He is also a member of the adjunct faculty at the University of Colorado at Denver, the University of Denver, and George Washington University. Helton is a certified management accountant, certified fraud examiner, and fellow of the Healthcare Financial Management Association (HFMA). He also serves on the HFMA board of examiners. A former health system chief financial officer, Helton has more than 20 years of experience in a variety of healthcare organizations across the United States.

**Francis G. Belardi, MD, FAAFP**, is a residency-trained, board-certified physician. During his 41-year career, he practiced family medicine in private practice, first with Kaiser Permanente Medical Group and later with the Guthrie Clinic. During his tenure at Guthrie, he served in many roles, including program director of the family medicine residency program; chair of family medicine; executive vice president for clinical affairs; and president and CEO of the Guthrie Clinic Medical Group, from which he retired in 2014. In 2006, in conjunction with King's College, he developed a joint physician leadership program that offered a one-year leadership certificate program and subsequently a master of health administration (MHA) degree. To date, 60 Guthrie physicians have completed the certificate program and 12 physicians have received their MHA. He has published several articles in the medical literature.